'This user-friendly self-help book is a must-have for teens and adults on the spectrum looking for evidence-based tools to help them lead happier lives.'

– Angela Scarpa, PhD, Associate Professor of Psychology and Director of the Virginia Tech Center for Autism Research

EXPLORING DEPRESSION, AND BEATING THE BLUES

A CBT Self-Help Guide to Understanding and Coping with
Depression in Asperger's Syndrome [ASD-Level 1]

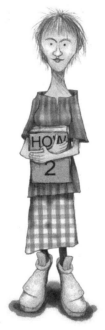

Tony Attwood and Michelle Garnett
Illustrations by Colin Thompson

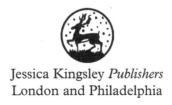

Jessica Kingsley *Publishers*
London and Philadelphia

First published in 2016
by Jessica Kingsley Publishers
73 Collier Street
London N1 9BE, UK
and
400 Market Street, Suite 400
Philadelphia, PA 19106, USA

www.jkp.com

Library of Congress Cataloging in Publication Data
Names: Attwood, Tony, author. | Garnett, Michelle, author.
Title: Exploring depression, and beating the blues : a CBT self-help guide to understanding and coping with depression in Asperger's syndrome / Tony Attwood and Michelle Garnett ; illustrations by Colin Thompson.
Description: London ; Philadelphia : Jessica Kingsley Publishers, [2016] | Includes bibliographical references and index.
Identifiers: LCCN 2016010238 | ISBN 9781849055024 (alk. paper)
Subjects: LCSH: Asperger's syndrome--Psychological aspects. | Depression, Mental.
Classification: LCC RC553.A88 A824 2016 | DDC 616.85/88320651--dc23 LC record available at https://urldefense.proofpoint.com/v2/url?u=https-3A__lccn.loc.gov_2016010238&d=BQ_IFAg&c=euGZstcaTDllvimEN8b7jXrwqOf-v5A_CdpgnVfiiMM&r=VCKr2NBFNTs4O_kp07esGY2J-doQEb4zTq5sCaeXa-I&m=VUpur47PjhtJUKVoc421FpqNV6ORtfKX3NDfTB2TiE4&s=Q8a9y0MuDUqLsqrnAYAwYRiqBwdpo3GZinQvlcaUI-o&e=

British Library Cataloguing in Publication Data
A CIP catalogue record for this book is available from the British Library

ISBN 978 1 84905 502 4
eISBN 978 0 85700 907 4

Printed and bound in Great Britain

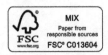

Contents

Exploring Depression and Asperger's Syndrome

There is a growing recognition among families and clinicians that there is an association between Asperger's syndrome and depression. The depression does not appear to be pre-wired, that is, an inherent aspect of Asperger's syndrome, but a legitimate reaction to the many adverse life experiences of those who have Asperger's syndrome. As clinicians, we have been concerned about the depth, duration and recurrence of depression in our clients at the Minds and Hearts clinic, and were determined to design and evaluate a Cognitive Behaviour Therapy (CBT) programme based on our clinical experience. The programme would also need to incorporate advice from a range of people: participants in the programme, our colleagues, and our friends and relations who have Asperger's syndrome.

We were also aware that there are some unusual aspects of the nature and expression of depression in Asperger's syndrome. These can include a difficulty conceptualizing and expressing emotions in conversational speech, occasions of brief but very intense despair, and a limited range of emotion repair mechanisms. The programme needed to be written in 'Aspergerese' – that is, in a style that would resonate with someone who has Asperger's syndrome – and be logical, structured and clear.

The programme evolved over several years, originally in the form of a manual for clinicians. However, we were aware that the key components of the programme needed to be incorporated in a self-help manual so that many more teenagers and adults who have Asperger's syndrome could benefit from the programme. We also needed to include aspects that would be only briefly included in a conventional CBT programme for depression, but are essential components for those who have Asperger's syndrome. The programme includes a range of activities for the creation of a positive and resilient self-identity and offers a new perspective on how we perceive and think about ourselves and our experiences.

If you have Asperger's syndrome, there is no doubt that you may have many reasons to feel depressed; however, you do not have to stay that way. The information in *Exploring Depression, and Beating the Blues* will help you better understand your depression, and, more importantly, teach you skills and strategies that you can use to manage anxiety and depression throughout your life.

PART ONE

Understanding Depression and Its Relationship to Asperger's Syndrome

CHAPTER 1

Why Does Someone with Asperger's Syndrome Become Depressed?

People with Asperger's syndrome appear especially vulnerable to feeling depressed, with about one in three adolescents and two out of three adults with Asperger's syndrome having experienced at least one episode of severe depression in their life. More adults than adolescents may experience clinical depression because the reasons for depression in Asperger's syndrome may intensify during the adult years.

The reasons people with Asperger's syndrome become depressed

Feelings of social isolation and loneliness

People with Asperger's syndrome have the desire for friendship, connection and social approval, but may lack the innate ability to easily achieve these outcomes. The result can be extreme feelings of social isolation and loneliness: as described by Debbie, 'the heartache of having unmet needs'. There can also be a tendency to over-analyze social situations and social performance, which can be exhausting and significantly contribute to feeling depressed.

Feeling rejected and not respected or valued by peers

The person with Asperger's syndrome may see other people as being 'toxic' to his or her mental health because of past experiences of bullying and rejection. These experiences have been described as giving intense physical and emotional pain. It is little wonder that many people with Asperger's syndrome choose solitude rather than company. However, as one of our clients with Asperger's syndrome said, 'I would rather be alone, but I cannot stand the loneliness.' Most people with Asperger's syndrome have experienced bullying, rejection and humiliation, and, without a well-defined and robust self-identity, cannot mentally counter what the bully says or cope with the social rejection and humiliation.

Many typical teenagers value specific qualities in their peers, such as the ability to make people laugh through quick wit, risk taking, being socially skilled, sporting ability and being perceived as 'cool'. Being popular is equated to self-worth. The qualities that a person with Asperger's syndrome brings to a friendship, however, might be loyalty, compassion, knowledge and open-mindedness, which may not be valued by typical teenagers. It is easy for the person with Asperger's syndrome to believe that their friendship qualities are inferior to their peers, and that perhaps, therefore, they are not as valuable as other people. This may result in feelings of low self-esteem, which contributes to feeling depressed.

Finding socializing mentally exhausting

Despite the lack of the innate hard-wiring for easily socializing, many people with Asperger's syndrome utilize their intellect to achieve social inclusion. Unfortunately, the psychological cost is high. The mental effort of intellectually analyzing every interaction to know what to do and say is exhausting. As a Buddhist monk with Asperger's syndrome said, 'For every hour I spend socializing, I need an hour of solitude to recharge my energy levels.' Energy depletion is a major cause of depression.

Internalizing and believing peer criticisms and torments

Frequent bullying and humiliation by peers can lead the person with Asperger's syndrome to believe that they really are defective in the ways described by the predators of the school and workplace. As Faye, a woman and public speaker with Asperger's syndrome, said, 'If you are told each and every day by your peers, your teachers and your family that you are stupid, you learn pretty quickly that you are stupid.' This can lead to beliefs about the self that are judgemental and critical, such as, 'I must be stupid', 'I am defective', 'There is something undeniably wrong with me', which can both make the person depressed, and keep them depressed. In contrast, typical adolescents, when criticized by peers, will have several close friends who can quickly and easily repair their emotions and provide reassurance and evidence that the negative suggestions are not true.

Focusing on errors and what could go wrong

People with Asperger's syndrome are very good at recognizing patterns and spotting errors, which is ideal when designing a bridge or analyzing an MRI scan of the brain, but not so great when thinking about oneself or the future. Being able to focus on errors or anomalies is a very important employment skill; however, when the person always uses this style of thinking when contemplating themselves or their future, depression may be the outcome. An example of this style of thinking is, 'I never get things right, I am hopeless, and I always will be'. There can be a relative lack of optimism; as the person with Asperger's syndrome achieves greater intellectual maturity, there may be increased insight into being different, with the resulting self-perception of being irreparably defective and socially stupid.

There can also be high expectations of social competence and an aversion to social errors and self-criticism. As Caroline stated, 'The worst thing about disappointing yourself is that you never forgive yourself fully', or Ruth's comment that, 'When something happens, such as not having your homework done, your inner voice blames and shames you for failing.'

Believing that change is aversive and unattainable

People who have Asperger's syndrome have great difficulty adjusting to change or the unanticipated, and usually actively seek and enjoy, and feel relaxed when there is, consistency and predictability in their daily lives. This can lead to a mindset that change is unpleasant and to be avoided. Another characteristic of Asperger's syndrome is cognitive inflexibility, which is not being able to conceptualize an alternative: in other words, a 'one track mind'. Thus, as described by Joshua, 'I may not want to change, know how to change, or believe that change is even possible.' This can lead to the belief that feeling depressed will inevitably continue and be consistent throughout life.

Not being able to cope with specific sensory experiences

An extremely difficult part of having Asperger's syndrome for many people can be the way they experience their sensory world, for example smells, sounds, textures and light intensity. Specific sensory experiences that are perceived by others as not particularly intense or aversive can be perceived by the person who has Asperger's syndrome as unbearably intense and painful. If the person does not have coping or escape strategies for avoiding or tolerating these intense sensory experiences, they may begin to feel very hopeless and depressed about how they are ever going to cope with this aspect of their life. The anxiety they feel while both anticipating and being overwhelmed by aversive sensory experiences can be paralyzing, and paradoxically, can increase their sensory sensitivity.

Being diagnosed with Asperger's syndrome

Asperger's syndrome is often perceived in our society as a disability or mental disorder. However, when we confirm the diagnosis of Asperger's syndrome in our Minds and Hearts clinic, the most common reaction from an adult who has sought the diagnosis for some time is tears of relief. Finally, there is an explanation for the differences that the person has been observing and analyzing for a lifetime. Now the explanation can be that, 'My brain is wired differently' instead of, 'I have a defective personality.'

Unfortunately, for some adolescents and young adults there is a rejection of the diagnosis due to genuine concern as to how it might be interpreted by society and especially by peers. There may be a sensitivity to the potential for being labelled in a pejorative way or associated with people with disabilities, which could then be perceived as official confirmation of being defective. Adolescents can also be acutely aware that peer ignorance of the nature of Asperger's syndrome may lead to subsequent rejection. The diagnosis and diagnostic label can become ammunition for verbal abuse: 'asparagus syndrome', 'hamburger syndrome', or 'arse burger syndrome', among others.

Family history of depression

We have known for some time that there is a higher-than-expected incidence of mood disorders, including depression, in the family members of someone who has Asperger's syndrome. Recent research has suggested that 44 per cent of mothers and 28 per cent of fathers of a child who has an Autism Spectrum

Disorder (ASD) such as Asperger's syndrome have reported having had a clinically diagnosed depression. In more than 50 per cent of cases, the diagnosis occurred before the birth of a child with an ASD. If a parent has episodic depression, then their son or daughter may have a higher genetic risk of experiencing depression themselves.

Having a 'sixth sense' emotional sensitivity

One of the diagnostic characteristics of Asperger's syndrome is a deficit in non-verbal communication: that is, the ability to read facial expressions, body language and tone of voice. However, clinical experience and autobiographies describe a 'sixth sense' ability to perceive and absorb negative emotions in others; the person is over-sensitive to another person's distress, despair, anxiety or anger, and this can occur without their actually seeing or hearing the other person. An example is a teenager in bed one morning, facing the bedroom wall with his eyes closed. His mother tapped on the door and silently walked into the room to open the curtains. He immediately said, 'What's wrong, Mum?' which was an accurate appraisal of her emotional state of high anxiety at that moment, yet he had not engaged the conventional, non-verbal cues to elicit that information.

The following quotes describe the experience:

> There's a kind of instant, subconscious reaction to the emotional states of other people that I have understood better in myself over the years. If someone approaches me for a conversation and they are full of worry, fear or anger, I find myself suddenly in the same state of emotion.

> I am able to distinguish very subtle cues that others would not see, or it might be a feeling I pick up from them.

Such is this sensitivity to another person's strong, negative emotion, the person with Asperger's syndrome can become 'infected' with that same emotion, yet be unaware why they feel that way. And because it can be so difficult to create a sense of detachment, many people with Asperger's syndrome choose to isolate themselves socially in order to protect their own mental health.

The duration and intensity of depression

Some of the characteristics of Asperger's syndrome can prolong the duration and increase the intensity of depression.

Self-reflection and self-disclosure

The person with Asperger's syndrome may have considerable difficulty recognizing, defining, conceptualizing and disclosing through speech their inner feelings to parents, partner and/or peers, preferring to resolve thoughts and feelings in solitude. They may avoid conversation about negative feelings and experiences, and try to resolve the depression by subjective thought or by using the special interest as a thought blocker. People not on the autism spectrum (neurotypicals) are generally more insightful, articulate, fluent and confident in disclosing inner thoughts and feelings. They are more likely to recognize that another person may provide a more objective opinion and comforting validation of emotions, act as an emotional restorative and be able to suggest an alternative explanation and reaction.

Neurotypical people may be better able to remember the good times and anticipate that similarly good times will be part of their future. This can be an effective antidote to pessimistic or depressive thoughts. Those who have Asperger's syndrome may have difficulty experiencing and remembering times of happiness and joy, other than the excitement associated with aspects of the special interest, and anticipate a life-long continuity of feeling sad.

Emotion repair mechanisms

Often, family and friends of someone who is feeling depressed may be able to temporarily halt, and to a certain extent alleviate, the depressed mood by words and gestures of compassion, reassurance and affection. They may be able to distract or elevate the mood of the person who is depressed by initiating enjoyable social experiences, or using humour, thus providing an infusion of happiness. Adolescents and adults with Asperger's syndrome can have considerable difficulty resonating with, or being infused by, the happiness of others. Thus, some emotional rescue strategies used by family members or friends may be less effective for people with Asperger's syndrome; they are more likely to try to solve personal issues by themselves, finding affection, compassion and others' optimism less effective emotional restoratives.

There may be one person within the family who takes primary or exclusive responsibility for emotion repair when the person who has Asperger's syndrome is feeling depressed. This potential over-reliance on one person can be concerning, as a mutual dependency can develop, and the person in the caring role can become both exasperated and exhausted.

Awareness of warning signs of a developing depression

One of the characteristics of Asperger's syndrome is a 'disconnection' between mind and body, such that the person does not seem to be aware of the internal physical and psychological signals of deepening sadness, such as depleting energy levels; or psychological warning signs or cues, such as increasing pessimism. One example of this is the case of a teenager who was recounting at the clinic his experiences of being bullied at school that morning. As he told the story, tears were welling in his eyes. As tears were about to cascade down his cheeks and were clearly visible to his mother and to us, his mother handed him a tissue. He looked at it in amazement and asked, 'How did you know I was going to cry?'

Another characteristic can be a delay in emotional processing time. An example is a conversation with a woman who has Asperger's syndrome who was describing a recent experience. As she was talking, with a voice that did not convey any specific emotion, tears started to stream down her cheeks. Michelle asked her why she was crying and she replied that she did not know the reason, but that after about two hours she would be able to process the events, thoughts and feelings and provide an explanation. This characteristic delay in emotional processing time can explain why someone who has Asperger's syndrome may have difficulty giving an instantaneous reason for having (or not having) a particular emotion, perhaps honestly replying to the question, 'How are/were you feeling?' with 'I don't know', which means, 'I am still processing and analyzing my feelings.' Thus, there can be a considerable delay in the expression of some emotions, such as grief.

The person with Asperger's syndrome is often the last one to recognize the signs of sadness or depression; these may have to be pointed out by others, with comments such as, 'You seem especially negative and self-critical today.' Without being able to perceive the early warning signs of increasing depression themselves, the person with Asperger's syndrome cannot take action, and is thus susceptible to the depression becoming deeper.

Vulnerability to extreme, intense emotions

In instances of intense depression and deep despair, some people – both neurotypical and those with Asperger's syndrome – may consider suicide as a means of ending their pain. This plan may be carefully considered over days or weeks.

However, in some people with Asperger's syndrome there is a difference in the way they come to this decision. They may experience what can be termed a 'depression attack'. Suddenly, without any warning signs to themselves or others, they experience intense, catastrophic despair and make a spur-of-the-moment dramatic decision to end their life.

These out-of-the-blue, extremely intense emotions are recognized in clinical practice, most often in association with an anxiety disorder and occurring in the form of panic attacks. The feeling of intense anxiety is sudden, overwhelming and unanticipated.

Depression attacks are similar, in the sense that there is no prior warning. The overwhelming despair may occur as a catastrophic emotional overreaction to what appears to be a relatively innocuous negative experience, such as making a minor mistake, being late or being teased. However, there may have been a backlog or build-up of despair over a long time that was not cognitively recognized by the person with Asperger's syndrome, or others. This final, simple event or trigger, releases the pressure that has been building for so long. The cap could not stay on the bottle any longer. The resulting conspicuous despair is very deep and genuine, and entirely unanticipated. There may subsequently be an impulsive action, such as jumping from a bridge, resulting in serious injury or death. Friends, family or colleagues who have been with the person immediately prior to this depression attack may not have identified any obvious signs that such an action was imminent.

We know that, should the person resist or be distracted from the impulse to act dramatically, the unanticipated, deep despair passes. Remarkably, in a short time, it gives way to a more balanced emotional state. For this reason, this programme includes strategies to help create a safety plan in the event of a depression attack.

Suicidal thoughts and actions

Recent research studies and reviews indicate that thoughts of suicide occur in 66 per cent of adults who have Asperger's syndrome. In contrast, the rate of such thoughts in the general population is 16 per cent. Research studies also indicate that 35 per cent of adults who have Asperger's syndrome have in their lives planned or attempted suicide. The actual suicide rate is unknown, but could be at least 7 per cent. Thus, the majority of those who have Asperger's syndrome have had thoughts of suicide, and around one in three have actually planned or attempted suicide at least once in their lives. This self-help book was written to reduce the depth and duration of your depression and thoughts you may have about suicide.

CHAPTER 2

The Nature of Depression

'Who are you?' I asked Henry, the very glum looking 14-year-old boy in front of me at the Minds and Hearts clinic, where we specialize in autism spectrum conditions. He looked at me blankly and some moments ticked by. Remembering his avid interest in cars, I rephrased my question.

'If you were a car, how would you describe yourself?' Henry thought for a moment.

'I am in good working condition', he said. 'There is nothing wrong with my engine, I have lots of fuel in my tank, the engine is running, but I am stuck in park, not in neutral, and I cannot seem to go. I receive a lot of care, people keep putting fuel in and I get serviced often, but it doesn't seem to make any difference. I can't go.'

Henry had seen numerous specialists for assessments, he was taking antidepressant medication and he had been seeing a number of psychologists for ongoing therapy. Despite these interventions, he had experienced little change over two years. He felt low most days, had difficulty both getting to sleep at night and staying asleep, engaged in few interests, never seeming to get very enthusiastic about anything, and experienced low energy. He found it difficult to get motivated about anything, rarely attended school, spending as much time as he could alone in his bedroom, and he felt hopeless about himself, his life and his future.

Henry was in the middle of a major depressive episode and his car metaphor was an inspired description of his depression. He felt that he *should* be able to function; he *should* be able to use his mind and body, and his energy; he *should* be able to get better with all the care and attention he had received. But the fact was, he couldn't. And the more he couldn't, the worse he became. He was extremely self-critical about not being able to get his engine into gear and get on with his life. He believed he was defective in a deep and unchangeable way and this belief, which he saw as a fact in his life, seemed insurmountable and unchangeable.

A major depressive episode

As you know, depression is a condition that is not easy to shrug off. Well-meaning people may say, 'Just think about something else', or, 'Just get up and do something!' Unfortunately, it just isn't that simple. We all experience momentary sadness, even feel depressed at times, but these periods of sadness tend to be transitory, and very soon we can put things in perspective and get back on track and feel optimistic and positive again. Deep sadness, or a major depressive episode, can persist over weeks, months, and sometimes years.

A major depressive episode may be diagnosed when a person experiences five of the following nine symptoms daily over a period of at least two weeks:

- sadness, emptiness, hopelessness and a sense of being a failure

- little interest or pleasure in nearly all activities

- significant weight loss without dieting, or a decrease or increase in appetite

- difficulty sleeping

- agitated or slow movements

- fatigue or loss of energy

- worthlessness or feelings of guilt

- difficulty thinking or concentrating; indecisiveness

- recurrent thoughts of death or suicide.

Henry had Asperger's syndrome. He also had a diagnosis of persistent depressive disorder, or dysthymia. This means that he experienced depressed mood for more days than not over a period of two years, as well as at least two of the above nine symptoms.

Bipolar II disorder

Some people who experience major depressive episodes also experience hypomanic episodes. A hypomanic episode is a distinct period, lasting at least four consecutive days, where the person is abnormally elevated in mood, extroverted, and energized or irritable, in addition to showing several of the following symptoms:

- very inflated self-esteem

- marked decrease in the need for sleep

- unusual talkativeness; a sense of pressure to keep on talking

- racing thoughts

- tendency to be very distractible

- increase in goal-directed activity; agitation

- increase in risky behaviours, for example overspending, investing in foolish ideas, or taking sexual risks.

A person who experiences both depressive and hypomanic episodes may have a diagnosis of bipolar II disorder. Bipolar II disorder can begin in late adolescence or throughout adulthood, though on average, it starts in the mid-20s. Bipolar II disorder is highly genetic, occurring most commonly among relatives of people with the disorder.

Managing a depressive illness

Whether the person is experiencing overwhelming feelings of sadness, a major depressive episode, dysthymia or bipolar II disorder, there will be significant distress and disruption to both their life and the lives of those who support and love them. The person commonly finds it difficult to attend school or university, find and maintain employment, or be emotionally available for friendship, intimacy or parenting.

However, it is important to understand that depression in all of its forms can be treated successfully. Initially, the main component of treatment is recognition and the measurement of the symptoms of depression. Please complete the following scale, the DASS-42, to measure your degree of depression, anxiety and stress. This will determine the level of depression you are experiencing currently.

www.depression-anxiety-stress-test.org/take-the-test

Once the level of depression is known, we recommend different responses and treatment, depending on its severity. If you have:

- *Symptoms of low mood or mild depression:* Utilize this book as a programme for alleviating depression, ideally with help from a clinical psychologist, mentor, counsellor, friend, family member or partner.

- *Moderate depression:* Make an appointment to see your general practitioner (GP) or physician to explore your personal, and possible medical, reasons for feeling depressed. Sometimes there are medical reasons for lacking energy and feeling sad, and the medical practitioner will arrange for tests, for example of the endocrine and immune systems, as well as discuss therapy options, including:

  - assessment and therapy from a clinical psychologist

  - utilizing this book, possibly in conjunction with a clinical psychologist

  - antidepressant medication.

- *Severe depression:* You must make it an urgent priority to see your GP and seek a referral to a psychiatrist or the local mental health care team, especially if you have suicidal intentions.

CHAPTER 3

How Does Depression Look and Feel for a Person with Asperger's Syndrome?

The majority of the clinical signs of depression in a person with Asperger's syndrome are the same as would be expected of typical individuals, but clinicians who specialize in Asperger's syndrome have noted other features that are specific to depression in a person with Asperger's syndrome. These features are described next.

Change in the special interest

The special interest of the person with Asperger's syndrome is often associated with pleasure and the acquisition of knowledge on an intellectually stimulating topic. However, when the person with Asperger's syndrome becomes depressed, the interest can become morbid, and the person may become preoccupied with aspects of death, perhaps almost obsessively watching movies that have a theme of despair and death. The reason for the change in the focus of the interest to the macabre appears mystifying, but is the person's attempt to intellectually explore and understand deep, negative inner emotions and express confusion, sadness and uncertainty about their personal circumstances. The morbid interest can be 'a cry for help', and an attempt to understand intense sadness and despair without having to engage in social interactions and conversation, which require the ability to be articulate and insightful with regard to inner thoughts and feelings. Parents, partners and clinicians may need to look beyond the focus of the interest and recognize a mood disorder that is being expressed in an unconventional way.

An indication of a very deep depression in the person with Asperger's syndrome is the loss of all enthusiasm for what was their special interest. Topics that once fired the person with passion, animating their conversation, creating energy and causing immense pleasure and relaxation, can lose value. When experiencing this deep expression of depression, the person is no longer interested in talking about favourite topics; aviation, entomology, Second World War tanks, Egyptology or whatever else previously captured their interest no longer acts as an effective antidepressant. Even the best-loved, most established interest may not have sufficient power to alleviate a very severe depression.

Anger as an expression of depression

Anger in someone who has Asperger's syndrome may actually be a sign of depression. People of all ages with Asperger's syndrome have described the functional use of anger to achieve solitude. When a person with Asperger's syndrome is sad or anxious they typically do not crave intimacy and connection with another person. Yet, if they express sadness, for example through crying, this is exactly what they tend to receive, by way of a close hug or close attention. They can quickly learn not to cry (someone will 'squeeze' you, and how will that help you feel better?), but instead yell or punch a wall, so that people will leave them alone. A person with Asperger's syndrome will often feel safer when alone, preferring time without interruption or distraction to process experiences and emotions.

Another characteristic of Asperger's syndrome is to have an explosion of destructive anger to 'cleanse the system', 'clear the air' or 'reboot the emotion computer'. As one adult said, 'It's a bit like wanting to vomit, knowing you will feel ill until you actually throw up. You get it over and done with and feel better. Getting it out of your system.' Thus, a means of recovery or repair for negative emotions is to discharge those feelings in an explosion of aggressive energy. A metaphor is having a severe, chronic headache (the sadness), which is quickly alleviated by a fast-acting pain relief tablet (the explosion of anger). In psychological terms, the explosion is a powerful negative reinforcer, and as such can become the person's preferred effective treatment for increasingly intolerable feelings of depression.

Thus, while we recognize that one of the typical key signs of chronic depression is lethargy and self-blame, psychologists also recognize that depression can be expressed as agitation and blame of others rather than oneself, using the term 'externalized agitated depression'. While the person is perceived as aggressive, the underlying emotion is actually low self-worth and depression.

A person with Asperger's syndrome may demonstrate many problems with anger and impulse control when feeling depressed, for example yelling for no apparent reason, throwing plates or a chair or punching a wall. These behaviours may be an expression of their depression, that is, their feelings of helplessness and hopelessness about themselves, the world or their future. Rather than 'surrendering' to the depression, they go into 'attack mode', becoming violent against a world (or people) that may not express acceptance and respect.

The person with Asperger's syndrome may not have a wide range of innate tools to communicate their true feelings as they arise; thus, these emotions may only be communicated once they are extreme, and expressed in a way that lacks precision and subtlety. Most people with Asperger's syndrome are not 'wired' to express emotion in conventional or subtle ways.

Alexithymia[1]

In alexithymia, the circuitry in the brain that is responsible for helping people to find words for their thoughts and feelings is not working as efficiently as would be expected, such that the person has a limited vocabulary of precise and subtle words for their emotions. As a seven-year-old child with Asperger's syndrome said, 'I need a language for my worries.' Alexithymia is a psychological construct to describe people who experience difficulty identifying and describing their emotional states and often occurs in people who have Asperger's syndrome. As Heather, a astrophysicist who has Asperger's syndrome, said, 'I do not understand why you need all those words for different emotions! I have two emotions: "OK" and "mad".'

This insightful statement raises a question: if somebody has only two words for their emotions, do they still experience the full range of emotions? The answer is yes. An emotion has four parts: thinking, behaviour, physiology and the subjective experience, or the feeling, of the emotion. People who experience alexithymia have difficulty with labelling, which is knowing the word or words to clearly and precisely describe the feeling. They will still

---

1   A Glossary of terminology which may be unfamiliar is included at the end of this book.

experience the thinking, behaviour and physiology of that emotion, but have great difficulty communicating that feeling in conversational speech. This is important to know, because people who have Asperger's syndrome may say that they are not anxious or depressed, but their thought patterns, behaviour and physiology will tell a different story.

Wearing a mask

Women, and some men, who have Asperger's syndrome are known to frequently 'wear a mask' to hide their true feelings and their true self from others, for fear of rejection. Masking emotions is a very intelligent and constructive coping mechanism, creating an appealing, but temporary, cure. As one woman said, 'I have done such a great job at pretending to be normal that nobody really believes I have Asperger's.'

However, 'faking it' or masking the real self and emotions in order to be accepted and liked can create a chronic sense of concealed alienation, loneliness and feelings of personal defectiveness. It can also be exhausting to lead a double life, significantly contributing to depression.

Suppression of emotions

Recent research has discovered that adults who have Asperger's syndrome are most likely to utilize the coping mechanism of suppression for strong emotions, rather than other coping strategies such as seeking support or putting the problem in perspective. Suppression of painful emotions can hide the symptoms of depression so effectively that the person 'slips under the radar' and does not receive the help they so desperately need. Unfortunately, the painful emotions do not go away, but instead intensify and elongate the depressive episode, and can also cumulate and lead to intermittent 'depression attacks' as discussed in Chapter 2.

Emotional dyskinesia

The considerable difficulty that some people with Asperger's syndrome have in expressing subtle or complex emotions in their face, body or tone of voice is known as emotional dyskinesia. This is not due to their masking or suppressing emotions, but to a difference in the circuitry of the brains of people with Asperger's syndrome. There is a mind/body disconnection, which results in some of the features typically observed in Asperger's syndrome: a facial expression that is sometimes described as a 'wooden mask'; a paucity of gesture; and a monotonic voice. Thus, the person may not look or sound distressed or depressed, so there can be a lack of recognition of that person's feelings and, consequently, access to support. As a result, the person may experience an increasing sense of alienation, and greater depression may occur. As one woman put it, 'People at school thought it was okay to bully and taunt me. They interpreted my lack of visible emotional expression as lack of feelings. They truly believed that I was not hurt by the taunts and severe bullying.' Unfortunately, it is still a common myth that people with Asperger's syndrome do not have feelings because of the lack of subtle variation in their facial expressions.

Difficulty understanding one's own emotions

People with Asperger's syndrome have difficulty reading the verbal and non-verbal signals that communicate emotions in others. They also have difficulty understanding their own emotions. Generally, we interpret our own emotions through being able to recognize both the internal (physiology, thoughts and feelings) and external (behaviour, physiology) signs of that emotion, and by understanding the triggers to specific emotions. A person with a non-Asperger's mind (neurotypical) is able to link experience with emotion fairly automatically, and so learns which experiences can trigger or cause a certain emotion. For example, we may very much enjoy the feeling of swimming: the enlivening experience of cool water on the face and arms, the feeling of moving, weightless, through the water, and the sense of calmness that comes with floating. If these sensations are recognized and experienced as being pleasurable, we may start saying to ourselves and others that we enjoy swimming and that it makes us happy. We have linked our experience (swimming) with an emotion (happiness).

People with Asperger's syndrome can have difficulty understanding that personal experiences are linked with an emotion for a number of reasons:

- They struggle to recognize internal bodily sensations and feeling states. If the emotion is not recognized, then that emotion will not be linked with experience.

- Due to alexithymia, emotions are not encoded verbally in memory with a 'tag' or label, thus they are difficult to retrieve from memory later.

- They struggle to reflect on and think about their own experience. This skill of being able to reflect on one's own experience is linked to 'theory of mind' ability, that is, the capacity to understand that another's thoughts, expectations, beliefs and intentions can differ from one's own: a sort of 'mind blindness'. It is now recognized that for people with Asperger's syndrome, 'mind blindness' applies to their own mind, as well as the minds of others.

- Their perception of the world can interfere with learning associations. For a person with Asperger's syndrome the world is often described as a kaleidoscope of sensations and experiences that are disconnected and confusing. There may be confusion about what is important to attend to; the feelings of self versus the feelings of someone else; and the overwhelming nature of certain sensory experiences that can cloud and obstruct all else. Unless the experience of the emotion is strongly negative, for example the intense primal fear associated with a snake, the link between the emotion and the experience can be lost in the myriad of other sensations and experiences.

The recognition of subtle emotions

Strongly experienced emotions may have a clear link with behaviour. For example, if their strong, negative feelings are linked with the experience of being with people, particularly new people and new social situations, people with Asperger's syndrome may make the decision to stay socially isolated. However, many emotions are far more subtle, and there can be enormous difficulty identifying, labelling and encoding experiences that link with emotions of happiness, joy, pride, self-satisfaction, sadness, relaxation, frustration or mild annoyance. When we are able to understand, experience and connect with subtle emotions, both positive and negative, it is more likely that we will be able to sustain well-being and happiness throughout our lives. Encoding and understanding positive emotions can allow us to relive those emotions through memories – an important way for cheering ourselves up during dark times – and also to recreate these experiences when we need them. Encoding and understanding subtle negative emotions allows us to pick up on emotions within us before they become overwhelming and difficult to manage, and can therefore be an early warning system for depression.

CHAPTER 4

What Type of Therapy Works for a Person with Asperger's Syndrome?

When you are to embark on a programme that involves new ideas and change, it is important to be confident that there is a good chance of success. The components of the therapy outlined in this book are founded on sound clinical research, as well as a combination of six decades of clinical wisdom and knowledge between the two authors.

Cognitive behaviour therapy (CBT) is currently the psychological treatment of choice for people who are suffering from depression. For example, NICE (the National Institute for Health and Care Excellence), a British government-supported organization, recommends CBT as the principal therapy for mild to moderate depression, and as an adjunct to medication for severe clinical depression. The *Exploring Depression* programme incorporates the components of CBT known to be most effective in decreasing depression. A description of CBT and a brief overview of the components of CBT incorporated within this programme follow.

Cognitive behaviour therapy

Cognitive behaviour therapy is an 'umbrella' term for a range of psychological therapies designed to treat depression, anxiety, anger and stress. There are also variations of CBT to treat relationship problems, schizophrenia, addictions, and eating and personality disorders. Each of these psychological therapies has some common underlying ideas, including:

- it is our perception or thoughts about events, people and situations that determine our reactions or feelings to them

- the consequences of our behaviours will determine how frequently and for how long we engage in those behaviours

- our thoughts and our behaviours can be measured and monitored, and change over time.

When starting CBT, the first stage is an assessment of the nature and degree of problems associated with a specific emotion, such as depression, using self-report scales and self-monitoring. Assessment provides you with an understanding of the causes of the problem and, to some extent, why the problem is still continuing and so deep. Initial assessment also provides a baseline with which you can evaluate the treatment programme.

The next stage is affective, or emotion, education to increase your knowledge of emotions within yourself and others. The text and activities help you examine the connection between your thoughts, emotions and behaviour, and identify the ways in which you conceptualize emotions and perceive various situations. The principle is that the more you identify and understand emotions, the more you are able to express and manage those emotions appropriately.

The third stage of CBT involves both cognitive restructuring to correct distorted conceptualizations and dysfunctional beliefs, and behavioural change to enable you to constructively manage emotions using a range of emotion management 'tools'. Activity planning and self-monitoring are an important part of this stage, and of the fourth, or last, stage.

Within the third stage of CBT (cognitive restructuring), the components identified by research to be effective, and so included in the *Exploring Depression* programme, are listed below:

- understanding and expression of one's own emotions

- identification of one's own thoughts and beliefs

- understanding and correcting distorted perceptions and dysfunctional beliefs

- increasing physical exercise

- learning how to relax

- increasing pleasurable activities

- use of social support.

The fourth, or last, stage of CBT is continuing practice of the new cognitive and behavioural skills in real life situations.

All four components are included in this programme.

Treatment components of the *Exploring Depression* programme

The *Exploring Depression* programme is a self-help intervention. Research indicates that the most efficient and effective way to incorporate a self-help intervention is to follow the programme under guidance, which means working through the programme mostly independently, but with some support given ideally by a professional therapist, such as a clinical psychologist, counsellor, or life coach, or by a friend or family member. This guidance should primarily be supportive and facilitative to assist you to take the steps recommended within the programme. The support may be given via face-to-face contact, telephone, email or any other communication method that you prefer.

We highly recommend undertaking this programme with the support of either a professional therapist, counsellor, life coach, friend or family member.

Research shows that for mild to moderate depression this guided self-help model is as effective as face-to-face therapy with a clinical psychologist, and has the advantages of being cheaper, more efficient, easy to use and more accessible for people who are reluctant to identify with experiencing distress, or are anxious that a psychologist will diagnose them as insane and they will be admitted to a psychiatric hospital. The programme will also be of value to those who live in rural areas with less access to clinical psychologists.

Even when there is access to a clinical psychologist, that psychologist may not have experience of, or confidence in, applying CBT to someone who has Asperger's syndrome. This book provides you and your support person with access to the necessary clinical knowledge base and experience of two internationally recognized experts in Asperger's syndrome, CBT and the psychological treatment of depression.

Understanding, identification and expression of emotion

A key component of CBT is understanding the difference between a feeling and a thought, being able to identify both within ourselves, and also being able to express our feelings accurately and effectively. Being able to perceive and express feelings and emotions accurately is an important part of being able to regulate emotions effectively. Taking the time to understand and express our feelings, even when this is difficult to do, is an integral step within an effective CBT programme. Stages 1–4 in the *Exploring Depression* programme largely focus on this step.

Use of structure and visuals

Research and clinical experience suggest that a person with Asperger's syndrome is happier and more relaxed when there is structure and routine to their day, and are also more likely to remember and implement therapy activities when they are regularly scheduled into their daily life. The *Exploring Depression* programme incorporates weekly planners throughout each stage to ensure that the activities known to decrease depression are planned and incorporated within your daily life. Practice makes perfect.

The weekly planners of this programme can be downloaded from the websites of both Tony Attwood and the Minds and Hearts clinic and can be displayed in prominent places in your home and at work or school.[2] These planners will serve as visual reminders of the important activities that are an essential part of the programme.

Self-monitoring

Behaviour and thinking changes can occur simply by starting to monitor behaviour and thoughts, without any other intervention. The *Exploring Depression* programme incorporates self-monitoring to assist with behavioural and emotional change, to allow self-reflection on which components of the course are working and which are not working, and to 'trouble shoot' and problem solve the barriers to success as necessary. This self-reflection is facilitated by an accurate record of what happened, rather than your retrospective perception (and possibly misperception) of events. One of the goals of CBT is for you to regain a realistic perception of yourself and the situation, rather than experience a pessimistic perception, distorted by depressive mood.

Physical exercise

Several research studies on the management of depression have found that physical exercise significantly reduces symptoms of depression. So beneficial is physical exercise for alleviating both depression and anxiety that some researchers have concluded that exercise can be used to manage depression

---

2   See 'Downloads for Exploring Depression' at www.tonyattwood.com.au or www.mindsandhearts.net

either as a 'stand-alone' or as an 'add-on' intervention or therapy. Thus, physical exercise is an increasingly recognized antidepressant. Unfortunately, depression can reduce the motivation and energy to engage in physical activity, creating a sense of lethargy. Added to this, people who have Asperger's syndrome may have felt clumsy since early childhood, which has led to the belief that physical exercise is a non-preferred activity, sometimes with memories of being ridiculed by peers because of a lack of agility. Nevertheless, as part of the *Exploring Depression* programme, regular exercise of some sort is encouraged, because of its undoubted benefits.

Pleasurable activities

A key component of successful CBT programmes for depression is to assist the person to discover or rediscover activities that they find pleasurable, and to increase their participation in these activities. In the *Exploring Depression* programme we have included the scheduling of a range of pleasurable activities from participation in the arts to being in nature or spending time with animals. It is important to create the list of pleasurable activities during a period of relative happiness, as when feeling very low-spirited or depressed, it can be difficult to remember or generate examples of your pleasant experiences.

Cognitive restructuring

Cognitive restructuring, a central component of CBT, allows the person to hold their own thoughts and beliefs as hypotheses about how things are, and then seek data or clear evidence to affirm or disprove their assumptions. In this way, you do not have to believe your first thought, for example, 'I am a failure', or 'Things will always be this bad'. Instead, you can carefully examine the actual evidence, as any good scientist or detective would do, to confirm or disprove your opinion. There is substantial research evidence that cognitive restructuring is an important component of CBT, but that it is not enough by itself to produce change. Research confirms that changing one's actual behaviour is also important. Hence, cognitive restructuring and a focus on behavioural change are important parts of the *Exploring Depression* programme. It is worth noting here that a common limiting belief for a person with Asperger's syndrome is that they cannot change their behaviour, experiences or circumstances. This belief is linked to a fear of change, even positive change. The *Exploring Depression* programme addresses these characteristics and encourages change for the good.

Use of social support

There is considerable research evidence to show that positive, supportive relationships with family members, friends and colleagues have a beneficial effect on both general health and psychological health. For the person with Asperger's syndrome, as discussed in Chapter 2, initiating and maintaining good relationships and social support with other people may be a specific challenge. In addition, other people may have been rude and abusive, causing an understandable avoidance of human contact.

Nevertheless, a person with Asperger's syndrome has a psychological need for acceptance and approval from others and for enjoyable social experiences. The use of social support is incorporated as one of the tools for decreasing depressive symptoms within the *Exploring Depression* programme. For the person with Asperger's syndrome, the social support may occur less often than for a typical person who is depressed, and the number of social support people may be smaller. It is also important that they are carefully chosen for their attitude and intuitive understanding of Asperger's syndrome.

Relaxation activities

Many people with Asperger's syndrome report very high levels of anxiety and stress, often in conjunction with depression. Bob explained that, 'Depression is the fraternal twin of anxiety. They play together in the mind, harvesting mental energy, stealing it from things we want to do and think.' We have noted in our clinical experience that many people with Asperger's syndrome do not recognize that they are in a constant state of high anxiety and/or stress, and they do not know how to achieve relaxation, a state of mind that seems so elusive. Being in a perpetual state of high anxiety and stress is mentally exhausting – and high levels of mental exhaustion lead to depression. Learning to relax can provide you with relief from anxiety, stress and depressive symptoms.

Consequently, we have chosen to include several relaxation activities in the *Exploring Depression* programme.

Self-awareness

In addition to the above components of CBT, the *Exploring Depression* programme incorporates activities specifically designed to increase self-awareness and mindfulness (self-awareness tools).

The term 'self-awareness' in this book refers to your ability to recognize and describe your own bodily sensations, thoughts, feelings, values and personality characteristics. By increasing your self-awareness, you will experience an increase in your personal strength and resilience. You may be considering these questions: How do I know that it is time to use a specific tool for emotion management if I cannot observe, feel or label emotions in my body? How do I start to challenge a poor self-concept if I do not recognize my underlying thoughts about myself? How do I design a life that will suit me if I do not know who 'I' am? This programme will address and help answer all these questions.

A common feature of Asperger's syndrome is a lack of vocabulary to describe feelings (alexithymia); we have also discovered another feature – a lack of vocabulary to describe personality characteristics (alexipersona). This will clearly affect the concept and communication of self. Increasing your self-awareness and ability to eloquently describe your feelings and personality, along with the other tools described in this programme, can enlighten and empower you to understand, manage, and eventually reduce, your signs of depression with increasing success and confidence.

Meditation

Perhaps the most powerful tool known at this time for increasing self-awareness is meditation. This can take various forms, such as transcendental meditation, concentrative techniques (making an object or the breath a focus of attention), Vipassana meditation, Hatha Yoga, Tai Chi, Qi Gong, guided meditation and mindfulness techniques (staying present to the moment). Whilst these tools for living are certainly not new – for example, meditation has been described in texts dating back over 5000 years – scientific research into their effects has only begun in the last ten years.

Meditation has now become an established psychotherapeutic technique and there are even specific therapeutic approaches that incorporate meditation: for example, Acceptance and Commitment Therapy (ACT), Dialectical Behavioural Therapy (DBT), Mindfulness-based Stress Reduction (MBSR) and Mindfulness-based Cognitive Therapy (MBCT).

Meditation becomes even more relevant to the person with Asperger's syndrome when we consider that each of the brain areas found to be positively affected by meditation are those areas that are known to be associated with the neuro-psychological profile identified in people who have Asperger's syndrome. For example, the areas of the brain that process sensory information, bodily sensations, thoughts and emotions, and those areas that allow concentration, attention, processing speed, working memory, organization and time management are commonly affected by having Asperger's syndrome, and it is these very areas that are most assisted by meditation.

The self-awareness exercises included in the *Exploring Depression* programme have been designed to increase mindfulness, amplify self-awareness and increase the effectiveness of the CBT programme. We regard these as an essential component of the programme.

Medication

Research on the pharmacology used in depression has primarily focused on serotonin, which is a neuro-transmitter in the brain. Increased serotonin levels have been associated with feelings of well-being and happiness. Serotonin deficiency has been suggested as a possible cause of depression, and medication can be prescribed to increase the levels of serotonin. The medication of first choice is a Selective Serotonin Reuptake Inhibitor, or SSRI. The therapeutic effects of SSRI medication may not be experienced until three to eight weeks after starting treatment, and it is not advisable to stop taking the medication suddenly. When the depression has lifted, it is important to continue taking the medication for at least four months to inhibit the chance of recurrence. Research suggests that the most effective treatment for severe depression is a combination of psychotherapy, such as CBT, and medication.

CHAPTER 5

The Perception, Learning and Thinking Styles Associated with Asperger's Syndrome

This programme is designed to help you understand and gradually reduce the signs of depression and gain new insights and abilities. It is important, therefore, that the implementation and application of the programme accommodate the unusual perception, thinking and learning styles including both learning talents and difficulties associated with Asperger's syndrome. This chapter explores those learning and thinking styles and aspects of sensory sensitivity, and describes strategies to enhance your ability to learn about yourself and feel less depressed.

The learning and thinking styles can include:

- intellectual strengths and weaknesses
- difficulty maintaining attention when confused or lacking motivation
- problems with organizational and planning skills
- one-track mindedness
- fear of making a mistake
- the need for consistency and certainty
- special interests
- alexithymia
- difficulty with self-disclosure
- a distinctive language profile
- sensory issues, particularly sensory sensitivity.

The programme is versatile, in that it can be completed alone or with guidance and support from another person, such as a clinical psychologist, parent, partner or friend. It can also be completed by a small group of people who have Asperger's syndrome, with one or more clinical psychologists as group leaders. Either way, the distinct learning style associated with Asperger's syndrome will need to be recognized and accommodated.

The inherent logic and rationality of CBT programmes help explain why we have emotions, and how to identify and measure those emotions, along with an exploration of new strategies to communicate and manage emotions, especially depression. This approach appeals to the logical, scientific thinking of someone who has Asperger's syndrome, who needs a rational explanation.

Concept of self

Our extensive clinical experience suggests that there is a component of CBT that is of relatively minor concern for neurotypicals (people who do not have Asperger's syndrome) but of great concern for those who do have Asperger's syndrome: that is, the development of a concept of self, or self-identity, as in the following quotation from a woman who has Asperger's syndrome: 'I don't know who I am, I cannot communicate my inner self with those I want to.'

During childhood and adolescence, a typical child has an evolving sense of who they are, their beliefs, values and personality. This requires considerable self-reflection, is built on and accommodates the comments of others, and includes reactions to personal experiences. There is also the development of an extensive vocabulary to clearly describe personality characteristics or traits. Our clinical experience has suggested that those who have Asperger's syndrome may lack a wide range of words or terms to describe personality characteristics in themselves and others. We have created the term *alexipersona* to describe this aspect of Asperger's syndrome.

A person with Asperger's syndrome may have difficulty with self-reflection (thinking about their own thoughts), due to the recognized characteristic of impaired Theory of Mind abilities: generally this has been taken to mean a difficulty perceiving, processing and knowing the inner thoughts and feelings of another person, but more recently, this term has been used to explain a difficulty perceiving, processing and knowing *one's own* thoughts and feelings. There may be a lack of ability for self-reflection; or there may be a hyper-self-reflection, to try to intellectually, rather than intuitively, decipher and analyze the thoughts and feelings of others and oneself.

Another factor affecting the concept of self is the effect of years of derogatory, critical comments from peers at school, such that self-concept is based on criticisms and rejection, rather than compliments and acceptance. There may also be a relatively limited vocabulary to precisely describe the more complex aspects of character: this is due to a recognized difficulty 'reading' people and determining their thoughts, feelings and intentions. Consequently, there may be a failure to form a schema (that is, a framework to enable future understanding) of the various personality types: this is invaluable in determining a match to one's own personality profile, for the development of friendships and relationships. The person may have had little to no guidance at school or at home on the vocabulary of words to describe personality types, nor any opportunity to explore and describe their own personality. We asked a teenager who has Asperger's syndrome to describe his personality. He thought for a while, and then said, 'I don't have a personality.'

We have found that the concept of self for those who have Asperger's syndrome tends to be very negative and fragmented, and a significant cause of feelings of low self-worth and depression. Thus, we will provide more strategies to improve your concept of self than would usually be incorporated in a conventional CBT programme, and endeavour to improve the vocabulary of terms you can use to describe yourself.

Intellectual strengths and weaknesses

People who have Asperger's syndrome have a different and clinically distinctive way of perceiving, thinking and learning, and tend to perform at the extremes of cognitive ability. Despite having an IQ (Intelligence Quotient) in the normal or superior range, they usually have a very uneven cognitive and learning profile on an IQ test. We have found that information from an IQ assessment can be invaluable in determining learning strengths and challenges. For example, if you have advanced verbal reasoning skills, with a relatively high Verbal Intelligence Quotient (VIQ) and recognized reading comprehension abilities, your understanding of the concepts and strategies used in CBT may be improved by the inclusion of recommended reading and by discussing the programme with others.

If you have advanced visual reasoning abilities and a relatively high Performance IQ (PIQ), your learning may be facilitated by visualization, such as visual imagery and practice in daily life settings. The phrase, 'a picture is worth a thousand words' is of particular relevance here. It is learning by doing rather than by reading.

Difficulty maintaining attention when confused or lacking motivation

Extensive research has confirmed that those who have Asperger's syndrome often have attention difficulties, which can include problems with sustaining attention when lacking motivation or confused, problems with paying attention to relevant information, shifting attention, and a tendency to be distracted by inner imagination (i.e. day dreaming). These characteristics will obviously affect the content and duration of many of the components of this CBT programme.

Other characteristics of Asperger's syndrome can be impulsivity and hyperactivity, which may be factors that you will need to accommodate during the completion of each stage. You may require support from someone to help maintain your focus and encourage you not to jump to conclusions, especially if the programme is being conducted in a home setting with many distractions. People who have Asperger's syndrome are more attentive to programmes that are highly structured, with short, discrete activities, and assignments broken down into smaller units, in keeping with the person's attention span. You may need to highlight key information; and the amount of environmental distractions should be minimized. Consider taking breaks between activities to enhance your attention and learning capacity.

Problems with organizational and planning skills

An associated characteristic of those with Asperger's syndrome in adolescence and adulthood is described by psychologists as 'impaired executive function'. This includes problems with organizational and planning abilities, working memory (especially auditory memory) and time management skills, as well as the ability to generalize information to new settings. This characteristic will obviously have an impact on a CBT programme. You may need an 'executive secretary', such as a parent, partner or friend, to help minimize the effects of impaired executive function. You will need to use the weekly planners and self-monitoring sheets as 'executive toys' and prompts to encourage generalization across settings; in other words, to help incorporate the therapy in everyday situations.

Due to the problems with generalization associated with Asperger's syndrome, practice in real life situations is an essential part of this programme. It is also important that the person acting as an executive secretary or providing encouragement is aware of the time you might take to cognitively, rather than intuitively and instantaneously, process and respond to social/emotional information. It is thus very important that they remain patient and do not interrupt while you carefully and thoughtfully process any new information.

One-track mindedness

A lack of flexibility in problem solving is a characteristic of impaired executive function, but is also a very conspicuous characteristic associated with Asperger's syndrome. The metaphor for this characteristic is that of a train on a singular track, representing a 'one-track mind'. Clinical experience has indicated that those with Asperger's syndrome are often the last to recognize and seek help if they are on the 'wrong track' and unable to solve a problem. They tend to continue using incorrect strategies, not learning from mistakes – that is, they fail to 'switch tracks' to get to the destination (i.e. find a solution).

This cognitive rigidity tends to become greater with increased anxiety and sadness. The inability to conceptualize an alternative response or strategy clearly influences the progress of a CBT programme. It is therefore important that you remember to be flexible in your thinking, by asking yourself, 'What are alternative thoughts, perceptions and actions in this situation?' It is important to remember, too, that strategies to improve relaxation can also be used to facilitate flexible or multi-track thinking. In real-life practice situations, try to spend some time calmly imagining alternative ways of perceiving, thinking and reacting.

Fear of making a mistake

A learning characteristic of Asperger's syndrome can be fear of making a mistake. When you are unsure what to do or say, and there is a possibility of making a mistake, the situation can become a trigger for you to engage a flight, fight or freeze response. Research on the learning abilities associated with Asperger's syndrome has identified a conspicuous tendency to notice detail and decipher patterns, and especially to identify errors. When combined with a fear of appearing stupid and being ridiculed by peers, this can have a significant effect on the ability to learn and to cope with potential mistakes. This can also contribute to feelings of low self-esteem, in that predatory peers can sense the vulnerability to this fear and tease the person, should they make a mistake, that they are stupid. This can eventually become a belief that they are actually stupid. Making a mistake is evidence to confirm that belief, and can result in a refusal to attempt any new activity that could end in failure: 'If you don't try, at least you don't make a mistake.'

In addition to this fear and dislike of failure, those with Asperger's syndrome are less likely to seek help, and tend to 'hit the panic button' when a solution is elusive. This can be an intensely unpleasant experience, more than would be experienced by a neurotypical person, and the person with Asperger's syndrome may give up prematurely, simply to end the emotional pain.

Over the long term, this pervasive fear of failure can lead to a need to be right, and a tendency to criticize and correct errors in others in order to feel good about one's own abilities. This is a form of psychological compensation, and criticism of others is used as a way of demonstrating intellectual prowess as a counterbalance to feeling incompetent and stupid when making a mistake. The sometimes pathological fear of making mistakes while avidly pointing out those of others can affect the development of friendships and team-work skills, which, in turn, can create feelings of sadness and low self-worth.

It is important that anyone assisting and guiding you to complete the programme should encourage any suggestion or attempt that you make. Adopt a positive approach to problem solving, thus implying that making a mistake or not knowing what to do is not a tragedy, a sign of intellectual disability or a character fault. People with Asperger's syndrome can be very sensitive to any indication of intellectual impairment, and some can develop a form of intellectual arrogance as a compensation mechanism. While arrogance is not necessarily a desirable characteristic, it can be used constructively. So you might think, 'What would be the most intelligent way to perceive this situation?' or 'What would be the smart thing to do?'; or you may consider 'If I stay calm, I will be smarter' or 'If I become agitated, I lose 30 IQ points, and my IQ will temporarily fall into the normal range.'

The need for consistency and certainty

People who have Asperger's syndrome seem to have a strong desire to seek consistency and certainty in their daily lives. They thrive on routine and predictability. They also often need careful preparation for unexpected change. It is important that there is a clear, visual schedule of activities for each stage of the programme, with information on the objectives and the duration of the activity. There is a list of activities provided at the start of each stage of the programme for this purpose.

Special interests

One of the central, indeed, diagnostic characteristics of Asperger's syndrome is the development of special interests. This can include collections of objects, such as rocks or spark plugs, information on topics, such as the life cycle of a butterfly, or an encyclopaedic knowledge of a topic, such as presidents of the USA or television programmes such as *Star Trek* or *Doctor Who*. The special interest has many functions: it provides feelings of enjoyment or euphoria in acquiring new items or knowledge on a specific theme; the intense mental focus acts as a thought blocker for feelings of anxiety, sadness or anger; it acts as an energizer when feeling exhausted or lethargic; and it offers a means of demonstrating an admired talent to others, thus improving self-esteem.

Thus, the interest can be constructively incorporated into a CBT programme. For example, thoughts of and engagement in the interest can act as an antidote to sadness, blocking depressive or negative thoughts, and infusing energy and a positive mood. If the person is having to cope with the negative feelings associated with being bullied and tormented by peers, or being set seemingly impossible tasks, a special interest in a character such as Harry Potter or Doctor Who can be used to provide an illustration of how a perceived hero copes with adversity.

The special interest can be used in the CBT programme to improve motivation, attention and memory. Conceptualization can be enhanced: for example, if the special interest is weather systems, the person's emotions could be expressed as a weather report, with heavy rain representing a low mood, a thunderstorm indicating agitation, or a clear blue sky denoting happiness or contentment. In the affective (emotion) education component of CBT, a project or field study for someone whose special interest is commercial planes, for example, could be to visit an airport to observe the emotions of passengers: the sadness when saying farewell, the happiness of greeting friends and relatives, and the frustration or anger in response to a flight being delayed.

Alexithymia

As discussed in Chapter 3, clinical experience and recent research have confirmed characteristics of alexithymia in the profile of abilities associated with Asperger's syndrome; that is, there is an absence of words to describe feelings, especially the more subtle or complex and interpersonal emotions. The affective education component of this CBT programme is designed to improve your ability to recognize and use the specific words to describe the various levels of sadness and despair, thereby diminishing the effects of alexithymia. An alternative approach, if the precise word is elusive, is to quantify the degree of expression of an emotion using a thermometer or numerical rating, perhaps from zero to one hundred, thus indicating the perceived intensity of emotional experience.

Difficulty with self-disclosure

People who have Asperger's syndrome have considerable difficulty describing their thoughts as well as emotions in a face-to-face conversation, that is, converting their inner thoughts and emotions into conversational speech. Although the person may have acquired, through the affective education component of CBT, a varied and precise vocabulary to describe a particular depth of emotion, there can still be considerable difficulty answering questions such as, 'What were you thinking at the time?' or providing a coherent and cogent answer to the question, 'Why did you do that?'

Often the reply may be, 'I don't know', and despite encouragement, there is great difficulty elaborating on this response. What the person is probably actually communicating is, 'I don't know how to grasp one of the many thoughts or feelings in my mind, hold that thought or emotion, then identify the word that precisely describes the thought or feeling, and then communicate that to you in speech in a face-to-face conversation so that you will easily and fully understand my thoughts and feelings.'

However, there can be greater disclosure of inner thoughts and feelings using communication systems other than face-to-face conversations. If an explanation seems incoherent or elusive, there may be greater clarity and insight if you type (e.g. an email or text message) rather than talk. There can also be greater insight into inner thoughts and feelings using music and art: for example, choosing a track on a CD or from an online media library that, through the music or lyrics, explains your inner thoughts and emotions; or selecting a scene in a movie; or writing a poem or story. Sometimes, creating a drawing, cartoon or collage may help to express the inner workings of your mind more effectively than a face-to-face conversation.

A distinctive language profile

There is a distinctive profile of language abilities associated with Asperger's syndrome. This includes:

- a tendency to make a literal interpretation

- a difficulty giving a coherent, logical and sequential description of an event

- a need for extra processing time for complex verbal information or concepts

- a tendency to appease by claiming an understanding when in fact the reverse is true.

For these reasons, the person providing guidance for you as you go through the programme should ensure that their speech is clear and unambiguous, and endeavour not to cause confusion by using sarcasm, double meanings or idioms.

They must be patient when it seems that your telling of an event or story seems somewhat confused or illogical.

They should allow you extra time to process any verbal information, and avoid unnecessarily long-winded explanations. They should not move onto new topics or a new component of the programme until you have confirmed that you have had sufficient time to absorb specific ideas, concepts and strategies.

If you are confused about anything, or need more guidance or clarity, be honest and say so. Admitting your confusion will not disappoint your guide, nor does it imply any lack of intellectual ability on your part; rather, it is an expression of wisdom.

Sensory issues

One of the diagnostic characteristics of Asperger's syndrome is sensory sensitivity. When conducting this CBT programme, it will be important to set the room up with consideration to light intensity, background noise, aromas, and the amount of personal space. If you seek sensory experiences in order to feel calm, the availability of sensory activities can help focus attention on the mental activity needed for the programme. Sensory activities might include manipulating a small ball of Blu-Tack, twiddling a pencil or gently rocking.

It may be advisable to engage in sensory soothing activities prior to reading and completing the activities in each stage, to prepare the mind for concentration.

Advantages of a home-based CBT programme

Conventional CBT is conducted in the room of a clinical psychologist over a designated time period of usually an hour, with between ten and 20 sessions. The advantage of this CBT programme being home-based is that the activities for each stage of the programme can be separated and conducted when the person with Asperger's syndrome has maximum motivation, attention and clarity of thought. Instead of having to complete all the activities within the hour, they can be dispersed throughout the day or week. The amount of time to complete a specific activity can be extended, if needed, allowing greater opportunity for both reflection and the exploration of examples and practical application in everyday life. However, it is also important to recognize and accommodate the problems associated with a home-based programme: for example, distractions, such as the television or computer, or obligations, such as domestic or family chores.

Advantages of a group CBT programme

There are advantages in having a group CBT programme, in that participants can:

- achieve a sense of belonging with a group of like-minded individuals

- develop friendships and mutual support with other participants

- rehearse specific abilities by using role play

- receive constructive suggestions from participants who have had similar thoughts and experiences, which may have greater value and credibility than the suggestions of the group leader.

However, if conducting the programme this way, there will need to be an explanation of the social conventions and protocol expected in a therapeutic group situation: for example, the importance of listening to each group member, taking turns to speak, and showing courtesy and respect for group members' opinions, even when these are different from your own.

In a group setting, there will probably be a mixture of 'verbalizers' and 'visualizers' among the participants, so that the style in which the material is presented and learned will need to vary according to each participant in the group. Impulsivity and hyperactivity will need to be accommodated, and can require that the clinician provides more vigilant supervision. The sometimes pathological fear of making mistakes, yet avidly pointing out other's mistakes, can affect cooperation and cohesion within the CBT stages. Rules of the group can include that there should be no malicious laughing or derision in response to a suggestion from participants, and that positive feedback and praise for constructive suggestions should be given. Our experience of running group CBT programmes is that participants who have Asperger's syndrome clearly benefit from knowing the group rules, and are sometimes less likely to 'break the rules'; in fact, they are more likely to enforce them.

Research on CBT to treat depression in Asperger's syndrome

The content of this self-help manual originally began as a group CBT programme designed by Michelle and Tony in 2012. The programme was recently evaluated using a randomized control trial in Brisbane, Australia.[3] Although only a pilot study of adolescents who have both Asperger's syndrome and signs of depression, the results confirmed that the programme achieved a significant reduction in DASS Depression scores (see pages 20–21 for a description of the DASS), with an almost 100 per cent attendance rate and a high proportion of participants reporting that they enjoyed the programme. This led the authors of the research study to conclude that they were cautiously optimistic that the *Exploring Depression* programme can help in reducing symptoms of depression in those who have Asperger's syndrome.

Michelle and Tony have also used the programme with adults who have Asperger's syndrome. Using the DASS, there was evidence of clinically significant change with some participants experiencing major depressive episodes at the start of the programme, but all participants scoring within the normal range for anxiety, depression and stress, at the end of the programme.

Thus, there is clear evidence of the effectiveness of the programme in a group format. This manual is an adaptation of the programme as a self-help manual to be completed on your own, or, preferably, with support and guidance from a clinical psychologist, or your choice of family member or friend.

---

3   Santomauro, D., Sheffield, J. and Sofronoff, K. (2016) 'Depression in adolescents with ASD: A pilot RCT of a group intervention.' *Journal of Autism and Developmental Disorders* 46, 572–588.

CHAPTER 6

Overview of the Exploring Depression Programme

Aims of the programme

While occasional sadness is something we all experience, depression is different; it is a deep sadness that can be difficult to break out of. The primary aim of this programme is to help you both understand and then gradually reduce your level of depression. It is designed to help you regain your energy, rediscover your enjoyment of life and appreciate who you are.

Description of the programme

The *Exploring Depression* programme starts with an assessment section followed by ten distinct stages. Each stage has initial activities designed to explain and enable the acquisition of new insights and abilities, followed by a number of projects to incorporate the new learning and abilities into your daily life.

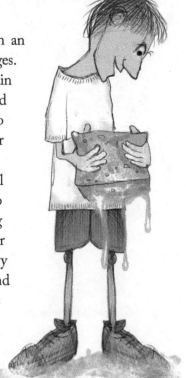

It is not enough to simply have an intellectual understanding about depression. For change to occur, it is necessary to apply that understanding in real life. To make this programme work for you, we ask you to make the commitment to try something new from the programme each and every day. Yes, there is work to do, but this is work for your personal benefit.

At the commencement of each of the ten stages, there is an overview of the objectives of that stage, a brief review of the material from the previous stage, and reflections on the projects completed during the previous stage.

We would usually conduct the programme at the Minds and Hearts Clinic in Brisbane as a series of ten one-hour weekly sessions with a clinical psychologist, as either an individual or group therapy session. However, as this is a self-help book, it is not necessary to complete a stage within one hour or within a one-week period. Some stages may take you longer to complete; there are no hard and fast rules. The programme is flexible to accommodate your personal needs and circumstances, and your situation and responsibilities.

If you find that you are not progressing through the programme at a pace of approximately three to four weeks per stage, or have completely stalled in the programme, we encourage you to make contact with your support person to determine if there are any barriers to your progress and to develop a plan to overcome them.

Overview of the programme content

Assessment

At both the commencement and the end of the programme we ask you to undertake three assessment tasks:

1. Complete a questionnaire to determine the personal reasons that you currently feel depressed.

2. Complete a scale that measures depression, anxiety and stress.

3. Create a list of your known strategies to reduce feeling depressed.

The purpose of these tasks is to further explore and understand your own expression of depression, and to establish a baseline measurement of your depression against which you can compare your results at the end of the programme, thus measuring the progress you have achieved.

Stages of the programme
Stage 1: Qualities and abilities

- Learn self-awareness tools.

- Identify your personal strengths, qualities and abilities.

Stage 2: What is depression?

- Increase your self-awareness.
- Understand more fully why you feel depressed and how it is that you stay depressed.

Stage 3: Tools to combat depression

- Understand the variety of tools available in an Emotion Repair Toolbox to repair your feelings of sadness or despair.
- Further increase your self-awareness.
- Choose your personal physical tools to combat depression or feelings of sadness.

Stage 4: Art and pleasure tools

- Understand the importance of expressing your emotions through art.
- Discover pleasure tools in the Emotion Repair Toolbox.

Stage 5: Thinking tools (Part 1)

- Explore the value of five thinking tools in the Emotion Repair Toolbox.

Stage 6: Thinking tools (Part 2) and social tools

- Learn more about thinking tools in the Emotion Repair Toolbox.
- Discover social tools in the Emotion Repair Toolbox.

Stage 7: Thinking tools (Part 3) and relaxation tools

- Continue learning more about thinking tools in the Emotion Repair Toolbox.
- Discover and acquire relaxation tools in the Emotion Repair Toolbox.

Stage 8: Relaxation and helpful and unhelpful tools

- Use relaxation tools for self-awareness.

- Discover other helpful tools and learn to recognize unhelpful tools.

Stage 9: A safety plan

- Be able to measure the depth of sadness and decide which tool to use at each level.

- Learn how to manage the most extreme level of depression, a 'depression attack'.

Stage 10: The future

- Imagine the sort of life you want in the future.

- Plan how to get there, using your self-awareness, strengths and tools.

- Review the programme.

CHAPTER 7

Assessment Before Starting the Programme

Before starting the programme, we need to assess why you feel sad and depressed, as well as the depth of your sadness. We also need to explore some of the repair strategies that you already know could help you feel happier. Information from the following three activities will also be incorporated in the subsequent stages of the programme.

At the end of the programme, we will be asking you to complete assessments 2 and 3 again. This will measure any changes in the depth of your depression, and also evaluate your increasing knowledge of what to do to reduce your expression of depression.

Assessment 1: Reasons why someone who has Asperger's syndrome can sometimes feel sad or depressed

There are many reasons why anyone can feel sad or depressed for a while. People who have Asperger's syndrome are more vulnerable to sadness and depression due to having more than their fair share of reasons. Here is a list of those reasons. Tick those that apply to you.

- ☐ Feeling lonely.

- ☐ Being rejected or humiliated by people at school/work.

- ☐ Being bullied and teased by people at school/work.

- ☐ Feeling exhausted from trying to be accepted and liked.

- ☐ Believing the criticisms of students at school or of work colleagues.

- ☐ Being sensitive to the suffering of others.

☐ Feeling exhausted from constant anxiety.

☐ Being aware of your faults and being a perfectionist.

☐ Taking corrections in school/work as personal criticism.

☐ Being bored at school/work.

☐ Not feeling understood by teachers/line manager/colleagues/friends.

☐ Not getting the school grades or work performance to match your intelligence or qualifications.

☐ Worrying about whether you will ever have a relationship.

☐ Worrying about whether you will have a successful career or career change.

☐ Believing that past bad experiences will continue forever.

☐ Feeling constant pressure to fit in and be like everyone else.

☐ Experiencing the loss of a friendship, pet or family member.

☐ Not being able to cope with intense sensory sensitivity.

☐ Experiencing too many changes in your life.

☐ Being diagnosed with Asperger's syndrome.

☐ Getting into trouble because of your anger.

☐ Not having enough strategies to feel happy again.

☐ Not being understood by your parents/partner or other close family members.

☐ Feeling invisible at school/work.

☐ Over-analyzing your performance in social situations.

☐ Being aware of and troubled by social injustice.

☐ Being unemployed or under-employed.

Any other reasons, such as emotional, financial or sexual abuse, or confusion regarding your gender identity.

_____

_____

_____

_____

Assessment 2: Depression and Anxiety Stress Scales (DASS)

The DASS is a 42-item self-report instrument designed to measure the three related negative emotional states of depression, anxiety and stress. The DASS has a series of statements, and you decide how much each statement has applied to you over the last week.

To complete the scale please go to:

www.depression-anxiety-stress-test.org/take-the-test.html

Add the numerical ratings for all the statements to obtain your total score.

DASS score: _____

At the end of the programme, we will ask you to complete the scale again to measure any changes in your total score that may be attributed to the programme.

Assessment 3: An imaginary scene

Imagine a scene where you are with a friend who is explaining to you how deeply sad they are feeling. You would like to help your friend feel less sad about themselves. What strategies would you suggest?

Make a list below of those strategies. How many can you suggest?

Suggested strategies:

_____

_____

_____

_____

_____

_____

At the end of the programme, we will ask you to repeat this exercise, and you can note if there has been a significant increase in your repertoire of strategies to alleviate feeling sad.

PART TWO

The Exploring Depression Programme

Qualities and Abilities

In Stage 1 you will learn:

★ about self-awareness

★ to identify your personal strengths, qualities and abilities.

Activities and Projects for Stage 1

Activities

- Self-awareness exercise.

- Identifying your qualities and strengths in your ability and personality.

- Understanding the value of giving and receiving compliments.

Projects

1.1 Identifying more personal qualities in yourself.

1.2 Identifying qualities you admire in a family member.

1.3 Identifying qualities you admire in a fictional character.

1.4 Creating a *This Is Who I Am* book.

1.5 Creating a compliments diary.

Self-awareness

As discussed in Chapter 4, increasing self-awareness is a very important step towards gaining a sense of calm and being in control of your thoughts and feelings, and for moving out of depression. With increased self-awareness of your own thoughts, feelings and bodily sensations, you are better able to respond to your own needs. Self-awareness is already within you to a certain extent, and the exercises in this programme will assist you to amplify this awareness so that it will be with you when you need it most. It is much easier to be self-aware when you are calm. However, it is when you are full of despair, stress, anxiety, fear and guilt that you most need your self-awareness.

The aims of the self-awareness activities in this programme are to assist you to stay mentally present during times of strong emotion, and at these times, to observe your thoughts, feelings, and bodily sensations without becoming too caught up in or distressed by them. Remember, you are not your thoughts or feelings or bodily sensations, even though it may feel this way sometimes. There is always a part of you that is observing these mental phenomena, and that part is not involved in them. This is the part of you that the self-awareness activities will assist you to strengthen. You may want to call the observing part of you 'the observer' or 'the true self'.

Self-awareness exercise

Complete the first self-awareness activity now. There are three self-awareness activities as accompanying downloads for this book. We will now use the first one, entitled *Bringing the Body into Awareness*, which will take approximately five minutes. The text for the exercise is in Appendix I. You can audio record your own voice using a digital recording device, or you can use Michelle's or Tony's voice on the download available.[4]

Remember that, even though regular practice will lead to a greater sense of calm and control, these self-awareness exercises are *not* relaxation exercises. If you do not feel relaxed during the exercise, then notice what you *do* feel instead. There is no right or wrong. The objective is to train your mind to place your attention where you want it to be.

You may find your mind becoming busy, and your attention wandering to other thoughts, bodily sensations, sensory experiences, memories, and feelings. Whatever happens, your task during these three- to five-minute exercises is to bring your focus back to the recorded voice and to observe what you are being asked to observe. This is the practice of mindfulness.

REFLECTIONS ON THE SELF-AWARENESS EXERCISE

Now that you have experienced the self-awareness exercise, write in the spaces provided your reflections on what it was like for you:

What emotions and sensations did you experience during the exercise?

_____

_____

_____

_____

---

4   See 'Downloads for Exploring Depression' at www.mindsandhearts.net and www.tonyattwood.com.au

How easy was it to maintain or regain focus?

_____

_____

_____

_____

Did you feel calm or anxious at the end of the self-awareness activity?

_____

_____

_____

_____

Identifying your qualities and strengths in your abilities and personality

ABILITIES

Everyone has particular qualities in his or her abilities. Are you proud of any of your abilities? Have you received compliments about them? This might include, for example, being an expert on a specific topic, achieving good grades in a particular subject at school or university, creating or repairing something, solving a problem, or being awarded a certificate at work. Or you may just know that you are particularly talented at something, such as having an outstanding memory for facts, being able to draw, sing, write or play an instrument, or maybe you have a talent in a particular sport or computer game.

While we are depressed, it can be difficult to acknowledge and appreciate our abilities and strengths. To help you with the activities in this section, try these tips:

- ask someone who cares about you or supports you

- think about when you were a child

- try to remember past compliments you have received

- try to remember past successes, however small.

List below your qualities in terms of abilities:

_____

_____

_____

_____

_____

_____

PERSONALITY

The qualities in your personality are those characteristics that describe who you are, such as being kind, helpful, loyal, resilient, non-judgemental, supportive, determined, trustworthy, thoughtful, honest, self-confident, intelligent, quiet, cheerful or generous, or having a sense of humour or a vivid imagination. These are just some of the many hundreds of words used to describe someone's personality. We have included more in the list of *Positive Personality Adjectives* (see Appendix II).

List below your qualities in terms of your personality. These are valued characteristics you recognize in yourself or that other people have used to describe you:

_____

_____

_____

_____

_____

_____

THE BENEFITS OF YOUR QUALITIES

Now think about how each of the qualities you have listed (in both ability and personality) can be an advantage in terms of:

- making friends and relationships

- self-esteem and self-identity

- enjoyment of life

- employment.

Make notes below on how these qualities are an advantage in each of these areas:

Making friends and relationships

_____

_____

_____

_____

Self-esteem and self-identity

_____

_____

_____

_____

Enjoyment of life

_____

_____

_____

_____

Employment

_____

_____

_____

_____

Share this list with a family member or friend, or the person giving you guidance in completing this programme, for their thoughts on how your qualities can be an advantage in your life now and in the future.

Understanding the value of giving and receiving compliments

Giving and receiving a compliment can help you feel happy, boost self-esteem and be an antidote to feeling sad. In this activity, take some time to remember compliments that you have received about one of your abilities or aspects of your personality that someone has noticed and admired. The compliments may have been given some time ago or recently.

What were the compliments about your ability?

_____

_____

_____

_____

What were the compliments about an aspect of your personality?

_____

_____

_____

_____

How did you feel, and what was the strength of that feeling, when you originally listened to the compliments?

_____

_____

_____

_____

How did you feel when you recalled the compliments?

_____

_____

_____

_____

Did you accept, enjoy and give gratitude for the original compliments?

_____

_____

_____

_____

One of the characteristics of depression is to not believe or accept that a compliment reflects a true quality. It is important to acknowledge that the quality that is being complimented is genuine, is part of you, and is appreciated by others, even if at this moment you have difficulty appreciating that quality in yourself.

Projects

The strategies we have designed and developed to enable your recovery from depression will only work if you think about them and practise them in your everyday life. To help you to do this in the most effective way, we have designed projects for you to complete between the stages of the programme. Some of them can be continued in your everyday life after you have progressed through all the ten stages. Following are five projects for you to complete before you begin Stage 2.

1.1 Identifying more personal qualities in yourself

When you are feeling depressed, identifying positive qualities could be very difficult for you. Discuss with your family and perhaps a friend or the person giving you guidance throughout the programme if there are more qualities that you have in your abilities and personality.

Make a list of these additional qualities in your abilities:

_____

_____

_____

_____

Make a list of these additional qualities in your personality:

_____

_____

_____

_____

1.2 Identifying qualities you admire in a family member

Is there someone in your family whose qualities you admire? If yes, who, and what are his or her qualities in abilities or personality that you would like to have in your own list?

_____

_____

_____

_____

1.3 Identifying qualities you admire in a fictional character

Is there a fictional character in a film, TV series or book whose qualities you admire? If yes, who?

_____

_____

What are his or her qualities in abilities or personality that you would like to have in your own list?

_____

_____

_____

_____

1.4 Creating a *This is Who I Am* book

Using a ring binder with plenty of blank pages, write at the top of a page one of the qualities that you either already possess or would like to achieve.

Then, at the top of each subsequent page, add another quality from your lists.

You can find all these qualities from the lists you already made in previous activities. Start with the qualities in your abilities and personality that you acknowledge, listed on pages 62 and 63. Also include qualities that other people appreciate in you (Project 1.1) and these qualities that you admire in other people (see Projects 1.2 and 1.3).

We realise that a ring binder is probably obsolete technology, and there may be a computer programme that you have on your computer or mobile/cell phone that will replace the function of a paper ring binder.

The ring binder, or equivalent, becomes a diary to record examples of when you expressed any of these specific qualities. The record can be written by yourself or another person, and can be illustrated by photographs and copies of grades and commendations. It can include a record of compliments from friends, family members and people you value in your life. Gradually, throughout and beyond the programme, you can add examples of the expression of your qualities in the *This is Who I Am* book.

When you are feeling sad, you can take out your *This is Who I Am* book and read and absorb the attributes that you have and are achieving, and remind yourself how people value you. This becomes an objective antidote to feelings of low self-esteem and pessimism, and is clear evidence of your qualities, thus encouraging a more optimistic and accurate perception of yourself and of your future.

1.5 Creating a compliments diary

Giving and receiving compliments can be a great way to cheer yourself up. Compliments can also cheer up other people and help you feel good about yourself.

Throughout the programme, decide each day to give two compliments. The compliments may be given to the same person or to two different people.

Create a compliments diary. Again, this can be electronic if you choose, or you may prefer a small notebook. Each day, record the two compliments that you give, and make a note about how you felt while you were giving them.

Also, when you receive any compliments, record these too. Note how you felt about yourself and what you thought as you received the compliments.

This project can improve self-esteem, help develop a positive self-image, and make other people feel happy too. Keeping a compliments diary is an activity you can continue even when you have completed the programme.

What Is Depression?

In Stage 2 you will:

★ increase your self-awareness

★ understand more fully why you feel depressed and stay depressed.

Activities and Projects for Stage 2

Activities

- Review of Stage 1.

- Self-awareness exercise.

- Identifying reasons for feeling sad or depressed.

- Measuring depression.

- Understanding depression.

- Personal energy accounting.

Projects

2.1 The Discovery of Aspie.

2.2 Thinking about thinking.

2.3 Writing in your compliments diary.

2.4 Creating and using a weekly planner.

2.5 Recording your activities on a self-monitoring sheet.

2.6 Filling in Daily Energy Account Forms.

Review of Stage 1

Write down some compliments that you received about yourself whilst you were completing Stage 1.

_____

_____

_____

_____

What were some of the qualities and abilities that you listed about yourself?

_____

_____

_____

_____

What did your family and friends add to your list of qualities and abilities? Did you agree with them?

_____

_____

_____

_____

What qualities would you like to acquire from a family member or hero?

_____

_____

_____

_____

Revise and review the reasons why someone who has Asperger's syndrome can sometimes feel sad or depressed. Which ones are relevant for you? (See Chapter 1 and Assessment 1 in Chapter 7.)

_____

_____

_____

_____

Self-awareness

Who are you? Answering this question accurately and positively can contribute to greater self-acceptance, and a feeling that you are worthwhile, as well as helping you to make wiser decisions in terms of career and relationships based on an accurate and positive sense of self.

As discussed in Stage 1, an important part of this programme will be increasing your self-awareness and sense of self-identity. The first activity of this stage of the programme is to complete a self-awareness exercise. Whenever it is time to learn new material, we will ask you to complete a self-awareness activity first. The purpose of this is to provide a pause between your other activities and engaging in this programme, and to ensure that your mind is clear and focused for the new material you are about to learn.

Self-awareness exercise

Self-awareness starts with an awareness of the mind and body.

In Stage 1, we focused on bringing the body into awareness. This exercise, which opens Stage 2, aims to bring the five senses into awareness. Certainly, many people who have Asperger's syndrome experience heightened sensory perception. Being able to cycle through the five senses, not dwelling on one specifically, in a three-minute period, will assist in being able to bring the five senses into awareness.

Once again, you can choose to record your own voice, using the text *Bringing the Five Senses into Awareness*, which can be found in Appendix III; or you can listen to either Michelle's or Tony's voice using the download that accompanies this programme.[5] The exercise will take three minutes, after which we will briefly explore its value.

REFLECTIONS ON THE SELF-AWARENESS EXERCISE

In Stage 1, you reflected on the self-awareness exercise *Bringing the Body into Awareness*. Take some time now to reflect in the same way on this exercise:

What emotions and sensations did you experience during the exercise?

_____

_____

_____

_____

---

5   See 'Downloads for Exploring Depression' at www.tonyattwood.com.au or www.mindsandhearts.net

How easy was it to maintain or regain focus?

_____

_____

_____

_____

Did you feel calm or anxious at the end of the self-awareness activity?

_____

_____

_____

_____

Identifying reasons for feeling sad or depressed

To be able to overcome your depression, it is helpful for you to understand more about what makes you feel this way. In Chapter 7, you completed a questionnaire about your personal reasons for feeling sad (pages 52–54). Have a look at your completed questionnaire now, and consider the relative weighting of each of these reasons in terms of how much you feel they contribute to your sadness. You will then know more about what you are dealing with, and the causes of your depression, which will enable you to learn specific strategies to overcome your sadness.

From the list on pages 52–53 choose your five most important reasons for feeling sad or depressed. Write them in the section below.

	Reason	*Percentage*
1.	_____	_____
2.	_____	_____
3.	_____	_____
4.	_____	_____
5.	_____	_____
	Total:	*100%*

Now, next to each of the five reasons, indicate the power of each reason in your life using a percentage, ensuring the percentages for all five add up to 100. (For example, being bullied and teased could be 30%, feeling lonely 50%, feeling constant pressure to fit in and be like everyone else 10%, feeling exhausted from constant anxiety 5% and sensory sensitivity 5%: 30+50+10+5+5 = 100.)

Are you surprised by the results? Sometimes there are no surprises, but just affirmation that there are certain aspects and issues in life that make you feel sad. Don't worry if you feel even more sad having completed this activity. Getting in touch with what makes you sad will often temporarily increase those feelings. Allow yourself to feel the feelings (where are they in your body?) and then continue with the next section.

What is depression?

Depression is a state of low mood and energy that can have a negative effect on a person's thoughts, behaviour, feelings and world view, as well as on their physical well-being. Depressed people may feel sad, anxious, empty, hopeless, worried, helpless, worthless, guilty, irritable, hurt or restless. They may lose interest in activities that once were pleasurable, experience loss of appetite or a tendency to overeat, have problems concentrating, remembering details or making decisions, and may contemplate or attempt suicide. Insomnia, excessive sleeping, fatigue, loss of energy, or aches, pains or digestive problems that are resistant to treatment may also be associated with depression.

Depressed mood is not necessarily a psychiatric disorder. It can be a normal reaction to certain life events (for example, grief for a person or pet), a symptom of some medical conditions (for example, chronic fatigue syndrome, underactive thyroid), and a side effect of some medical treatments (for example, Roacutane for acne, stimulants to treat ADHD).

Signs of depression

Common characteristics or signs associated with depression include:

- moodiness that is out of character

- increased irritability and frustration

- difficulty accepting minor personal criticisms

- tendency to spend less time with friends and family

- loss of interest in food, sexual activity, exercise or other pleasurable activities

- wakefulness throughout the night

- preference for staying home from school, college, university or work

- increase in physical health complaints such as fatigue, pain and digestive problems

- slowing down of thoughts and actions

- feelings of deep sadness that last for more than two weeks

- frequent feelings of:
  - helplessness
  - apathy
  - anxiety
  - 'emptiness'
  - hopelessness
  - guilt
- poor concentration
- difficulty making decisions
- tendency to contemplate the potential benefits of suicide
- not caring about others or yourself
- preoccupation with gloomy thoughts
- tendency to be critical of your own abilities
- difficulty enjoying and resonating with the happiness of others.

Measuring depression

Measuring depression can be helpful, because different strategies can work at different levels of depression. It is also helpful to understand how each level of depression feels in our bodies so that we can be more aware of the lower levels of depression, and in that way get to intervene earlier rather than later.

Below is a 'thermometer' to measure the 'temperature' (that is, the depth or intensity) of feeling sad.

On the left of the thermometer are the words to describe the different levels of intensity. You may want to add words or change them to words that you are more likely to use.

On the right of the thermometer are spaces for you to write down the different reasons for your own sadness or depression, corresponding to the level of depression or sadness they can trigger.

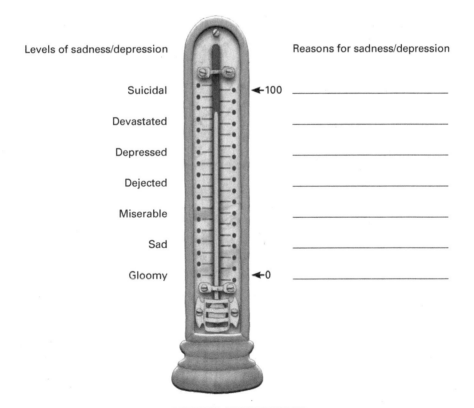

SADNESS THERMOMETER

Why do we stay depressed?

Did you know that life circumstances are actually only one small part of why we feel happy or sad?

Research has shown that everyone has a 'set point' or default level for happiness. There have been many studies conducted to understand why people feel happy, sad or depressed. One of the reasons is that we were born that way. Our genes are a significant contributor to how we are feeling from day to day. But it is not the whole story. Most of us tend to think that we feel a certain way because of something that happened to us, that is, our life circumstances: for example, being poor or rich, healthy or ill, popular or unpopular, having two parents or one. However, surprisingly, research shows us that life circumstances account for a very small part of how we feel. In fact, the biggest factors, apart from our genes, in influencing how we feel, are our own thoughts or attitudes, and our actions.

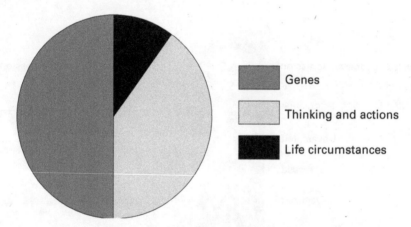

FACTORS INFLUENCING OUR FEELINGS

If we look at the simple diagram below, we can understand that the way we feel is a cycle. We are born with a particular set-point for happiness. Our brain gives us information about how to think and feel, which in turn determines what we do, for example, whether we exercise, make goals for the day, stay in bed, avoid people, etc. What we do determines what happens to us, that is, our outcomes, and these outcomes feed information back to the brain, and the cycle continues.

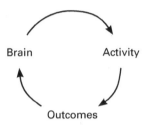

Brain

Activity

Outcomes

THE CYCLE OF EMOTIONS

In depression, the cycle usually looks something like this:

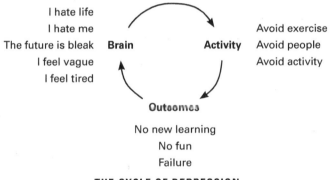

I hate life
I hate me
The future is bleak
I feel vague
I feel tired

Brain

Activity

Avoid exercise
Avoid people
Avoid activity

Outcomes

No new learning
No fun
Failure

THE CYCLE OF DEPRESSION

Understanding depression

UNDERSTANDING YOUR OWN CYCLE OF DEPRESSION

Consider your own thoughts, feelings and activity when you are depressed. Write your observations in the spaces below:

What thoughts do you have when you feel depressed?

_____

_____

_____

_____

What feelings do you have when you are depressed?

_____

_____

_____

_____

What do you do when you are depressed?

_____

_____

_____

_____

What do you not do when you are depressed?

_____

_____

_____

_____

UNDERSTANDING THE CONTRIBUTION OF ASPERGER'S SYNDROME TO YOUR MOOD

You may feel that your diagnosis of Asperger's syndrome contributes to the way you feel, both positively and negatively. Consider these factors now, and answer the following questions.

Does having Asperger's syndrome contribute to you feeling sad or depressed? If yes, how?

_____

_____

_____

_____

Does having Asperger's syndrome give you any positive qualities and experiences?

_____

_____

_____

_____

Energy accounting

Maja Toudal from Denmark has Asperger's syndrome, and she originally created the concept of energy accounting to help her identify situations that could be psychologically 'toxic' and contribute to her feeling depressed. She wanted to create positive change and cope with her cycles of depression. A part of this concept has been modified for this programme to help you overcome depression.

One of the causes and characteristics of sadness and depression is long-term energy depletion. It is as though you have an energy bank account; throughout the day there are both withdrawals and deposits of energy, as suggested in the following lists:

Energy withdrawals:

- Socializing
- Change in routine or expectations
- Making a mistake
- Sensory sensitivity
- Coping with anxiety
- Negative thoughts
- Crowds
- Being teased or excluded
- Sensitivity to other people's moods
- Over-analyzing social performance

Energy deposits:

- Solitude
- Special interest
- Physical activity
- Animals and nature
- Computer games
- Sleep
- Drawing/being creative
- Reading
- Listening to music
- Favourite food

These suggestions would be quite typical for a person with Asperger's syndrome. However, for someone who does not have Asperger's syndrome, the withdrawals and deposits would probably be very different; for example, socializing and changes to routines and expectations may, for some neurotypical people, be perceived as exciting and energizing, and thus be included in the deposit column.

Personal energy accounting

PART I: WITHDRAWALS AND DEPOSITS

In the table below, make a list of the typical daily withdrawals and deposits of energy in your life in the activity/experience columns.

LEDGER ENERGY ACCOUNT			
Withdrawals		**Deposits**	
Activity/Experience	(0–100)	Activity/Experience	(0–100)

PART 2: ENERGY RANGE OF WITHDRAWALS AND DEPOSITS

With energy accounting, we need a form of 'currency', that is, a numerical measure or value of how much an activity or experience drains or refreshes our energy from day to day.

The second part of this activity is to rate, from 0–100, the energy range of each activity or experience in your withdrawal or deposit columns. For example, on some days, socializing can drain you of energy at a value of around 20, but on other days it could be 100. The entry in the ledger above would therefore be 20–100. In the deposit column, on some days, listening to music would have an energizing value of 15, while on other days, a value of 40. Thus, the entry in the ledger would be 15–40.

PART 3: DAILY ENERGY ACCOUNTING

For this part of the activity, you will need to use a Daily Energy Account Form, which you will find in Appendix IV. Now you will apply the concept of energy accounting to your experiences on a particular day. List the specific activities or experiences that were either an energy withdrawal or deposit yesterday. Write the value (that is, a single score between 0 and 100) of each of these activities to measure how draining or energizing they were.

Then add all the numerical values in each of the two columns to see if your energy bank balance at the end of yesterday was in debit or credit – that is, in the black or in the red.

If your account was in the black, with more deposits than withdrawals, this is good energy accounting, and you will have reserves in your energy bank account to cope with subsequent energy draining experiences over the next few days.

If the account is in the red, however, with more withdrawals than deposits, you will need to achieve more energy 'income' tomorrow or over the next few days. If you do not achieve a 'healthy' energy bank balance, the lack of energy in your account will increase the depth and duration of your lethargy and depression.

Over the duration of this programme, you may be able to reduce the value of the energy withdrawals, learn strategies to stop 'spending' and increase the value and range of the energy deposits, using the activities to be described within the concept of an Emotion Repair Toolbox.

Projects

There now follows some reading and activities for you to complete before you begin Stage 3 of the programme. As discussed at the end of Stage 1, it is essential to complete the projects even when you may not feel like it. As you know, it is often the case that we have to actively do things to give ourselves more energy in order to feel better, rather than waiting until we feel better in order to be able to do things.

2.1 The Discovery of Aspie

Read the following article and answer the questions at the end.

The Discovery of Aspie
By Carol Gray and Tony Attwood

Some of the best discoveries of modern times were creative and determined efforts to answer 'What if...?' questions. What if people could fly? What if electrical energy could be harnessed to produce light? What if there was an easily accessible, international communication and information network? The answers have resulted in permanent changes: air travel, light bulbs, the Internet. These discoveries have rendered their less effective counterparts practically extinct: gone are the stagecoach, gas lighting, and multi-volume hardbound encyclopaedias. These improvements remind us of our option and ability to experiment, re-mould, re-think, and imagine. In that spirit, we propose a new question: What if Asperger's syndrome was defined by its strengths? What changes might occur?

Moving from diagnosis to discovery

Making any diagnosis requires attention to weaknesses, the observation and interpretation of signs and symptoms that vary from typical development or health. Certainly, it would be a little disarming to visit a doctor for a diagnosis, only to have her inquire, 'So, what feels absolutely great?'

The DSM-5 (American Psychiatric Association 2013) assists in the identification of a variety of mental disorders. It is used by psychiatrists and clinical psychologists to match observed weaknesses, symptoms and behaviours to text. In the DSM-5, Autism Spectrum Disorder, such as Asperger's syndrome, is identified by specific diagnostic criteria, a constellation of observed social communication characteristics and behaviours. Once diagnosed, a child or adult with the diagnosis is referred to as a person with an Autism Spectrum Disorder such as Asperger's syndrome.

Unlike 'diagnosis,' the term 'discovery' often refers to the identification of a person's strengths or talents. Actors are discovered. Artists and musicians are discovered. A great friend is discovered. These people are identified by an informal combination of evaluation and awe that ultimately concludes that this person – more than most others – possesses admirable qualities, abilities, and/or talents. It's an acknowledgment that, '...you know, he's better than me at...' In referring to people with respect to their talents or abilities, diagnostic terminology is not required; labels like musician, artist, or poet are welcomed and considered complimentary.

If Asperger's syndrome was identified by observation of strengths and talents, it would no longer be in the DSM-5, nor would it be referred to as a syndrome. After all, a reference to someone with special strengths or talents does not use terms with negative connotations (it's artist and poet, not Artistically Arrogant or Poetically Preoccupied), nor does it attach someone's proper name to the word 'syndrome' (it's vocalist or soloist, not Sinatra's Syndrome).

New ways of thinking often lead to discoveries that consequently discard their outdated predecessors. It could result in typical people rethinking their responses and rescuing a missed opportunity to take advantage of the contribution of those with Asperger's syndrome to culture and knowledge.

Discovery criteria for Asperger's syndrome by Attwood and Gray

A. A qualitative advantage in social communication and social interaction, across multiple contexts, as manifested by a majority of the following, currently or by history:

  1. peer relationships characterized by absolute loyalty and impeccable dependability

  2. freedom from sexism, 'ageism', or cultural or social status biases; ability to regard others at 'face value'

3. speaking one's mind irrespective of social context or adherence to personal beliefs

4. ability to pursue personal theory or perspective despite conflicting evidence

5. seeking an audience or friends capable of: enthusiasm for unique interests and topics; consideration of details; spending time discussing a topic that may not be of primary interest to others

6. listening without continual judgement or assumption

7. interest primarily in significant contributions to conversation; preferring to avoid 'ritualistic small talk' or socially trivial statements and superficial conversation

8. seeking sincere, positive, genuine friends with an intelligent sense of humour.

ALSO: Fluent in Aspergerese, a social language characterized by at least three of the following:

1. a determination to seek the truth

2. conversation free of hidden meaning or agenda

3. advanced vocabulary and interest in words

4. fascination with word-based humour, such as puns

5. advanced use of pictorial metaphor.

B. Cognitive skills characterized by at least four of the following:

1. strong preference for detail

2. original, often unique perspective in problem solving

3. exceptional memory and/or recall of details often forgotten or disregarded by others, for example: names, dates, schedules, routines

4. avid perseverance in gathering and cataloguing information on a topic of interest

5. persistence of thought

6. encyclopaedic or digital knowledge of one or more topics

7. knowledge of routines and a focused desire to maintain order, consistency and accuracy

8. clarity of values/decision making unaltered by social, political or financial factors

9. acute sensitivity to specific sensory experiences and stimuli, for example: hearing, touch, vision, and/or smell.

C. Additional possible features:

1. strength in individual sports and games, particularly those involving endurance, visual accuracy or intellect, including rowing, swimming, bowling, chess

2. 'social unsung hero' with trusting optimism: frequent victim of prejudices and predatory behaviour of others, while steadfast in the belief of the possibility of genuine friendship

3. increased probability over general population of attending university after high school

4. often take care of others outside the range of typical development.

Perhaps we have discovered the next stage of human evolution?

Ask those who support you and are important in your life to also read the article. Discuss the article with them. What do you think about the article? Was it helpful and why? What did other people think about it? Write your and their comments in the section below.

_____

_____

_____

_____

_____

_____

_____

2.2 Thinking about thinking

Think of a time during the last week when you felt happy. What were your happy thoughts?

_____

_____

_____

_____

How happy were you from 0 to 100? _____

Think of a time during the last week when you felt sad. What were your sad thoughts?

_____

_____

_____

_____

How sad were you? Use the sadness thermometer on page 79 to help you to measure your sadness from 0 to 100 _____

2.3 Writing in your compliments diary

Continue to write into your compliments diary both the two compliments you give each day, and any that you receive. Note how you feel about both giving and receiving these compliments.

2.4 Creating and using a weekly planner

You have now learned and practised a self-awareness exercise that helps you 'get in touch' with your senses. This is a really important step towards being able to manage your strong emotions. Doing this regularly will increase your sense of feeling calm and in control.

Look at the weekly planner for Stage 2. You can download this or photocopy it. First, fill in on the planner the activities to which you are committed (work, study, domestic chores, appointments etc.).

Next, make a note for each day when you will fit in the three- or five-minute self-awareness exercise. It might, for example, be best to do it last thing at night when you are in bed; or it may be easier to do the exercise first thing in the morning; or perhaps you will find it easier to do during a natural break in your day, for example at morning tea or lunch. To make this decision, it is helpful to visualize yourself doing the exercise: Where will you sit or lie? Who will be around? How will you get privacy to practise it? When you have established what will work for you, write your five-minute daily exercise onto your weekly planner.

WEEKLY PLANNER STAGE 2		
Morning	**Afternoon**	**Evening**
Monday		
Tuesday		
Wednesday		
Thursday		
Friday		
Saturday		
Sunday		
Schedule: Self-awareness exercise (daily)		

2.5 Recording your activities on a self-monitoring sheet

Each time you practise the self-awareness exercise, make a note on the self-monitoring sheet on the next page, noting in the column provided how you felt both during and after the exercise.

This is helpful, as physically recording the time and making notes about your observations is a scientific way to understand and change behaviour.

Ensure the self-monitoring sheet is clearly visible, in a place that you look on a daily basis. If you know yourself to be forgetful, use an additional strategy to help you remember to record your observations. For example, place a rubber band around your wrist so that each time you notice the band, you will be reminded about doing your self-monitoring at the designated time; or you may programme your computer or phone to remind you.

SELF-MONITORING STAGE 2	
Self-awareness exercise	What I noticed
Monday	
Tuesday	
Wednesday	
Thursday	
Friday	
Saturday	
Sunday	

2.6 Filling in Daily Energy Account Forms

Between this and the next stage of the programme, duplicate and complete several Daily Energy Account Forms (Appendix IV). See if there is a pattern developing. Is there a risk of an imminent 'energy crash', or are you maintaining a healthy energy bank balance?

This activity can also help you identify when in the day or week you have the most energy, and thus when you may be more able to complete some of the activities in this programme.

Tools to Combat Depression

In Stage 3 you will:

★ learn about the variety of tools available in an Emotion Repair Toolbox to help repair your feelings of despair

★ discover more self-awareness tools

★ choose physical tools that you can start using from today as an antidote to depression or feelings of sadness.

Activities and Projects for Stage 3

Activities

• Review of Stage 2.

• Self-awareness exercise.

• Identifying your own physical tools.

Projects

3.1 Writing in your compliments diary.

3.2 Adding regular physical exercise to your weekly planner.

3.3 Recording your activity on your self-monitoring sheet.

Review of Stage 2

THE REASONS FOR FEELING DEPRESSED

How can the things we do contribute to depression?

_____

_____

_____

_____

How can our thoughts contribute to depression?

_____

_____

_____

COMPLIMENTS

Did you remember to give two compliments each day? How did giving these compliments affect your mood?

_____

_____

_____

_____

REFLECTIONS ON STAGE 2 PROJECTS

What have your happy thoughts been since you completed Stage 2?

_____

_____

_____

_____

What have been your sad thoughts?

_____

_____

_____

_____

What did you think about the Discovery of Aspie article?

_____

_____

_____

_____

Which qualities of Aspie did you relate to?

_____

_____

_____

_____

Self-awareness exercise

Complete the three-minute exercise, *Bringing the Five Senses into Awareness* (see Appendix III). This will refresh and prepare your mind for the new information and activities that follow.

The advantages of Asperger's syndrome

People who have Asperger's syndrome have different (but not defective) ways of perceiving the world, learning, and achieving success. This success is often achieved in those areas of talent particularly associated with Asperger's syndrome, such as expertise on a particular topic, originality in problem solving, creativity in the arts, and exceptional kindness and compassion.

The pleasures in life for someone with Asperger's syndrome can also be different but intensely enjoyable, such as a special interest or talent, having a natural ability to understand and relate to animals, or achieving the higher levels of computer games.

Most of the great advances in the sciences, arts and humanities have been made by people who have or had the characteristics of Asperger's syndrome. As Temple Grandin said, 'If the world was left to you socialites, we would still be in caves, talking to each other.' The world will always need such people.

Here are some illustrious people who have been considered as having the characteristics of Asperger's syndrome. Those characteristics may well have made a significant contribution to their achievements:

Hans Christian Andersen	Bobby Fischer	Stephen King
Jane Austen	Temple Grandin	Stanley Kubrick
Dan Aykroyd	Benny Hill	Isaac Newton
Susan Boyle	Alfred Hitchcock	Gary Numan
David Byrne	Howard Hughes	Tim Page
Thomas Edison	Thomas Jefferson	B.F. Skinner
Albert Einstein	Carl Jung	Andy Warhol

The Emotion Repair Toolbox

There are specific, effective strategies to help repair feelings of depression and sadness. These strategies, such as physical exercise or engaging in enjoyable hobbies, are examples of what will now be referred to as 'tools', and their function is as follows:

- Self-awareness tools: for self-regulation and clarity of thought.

- Physical tools: for well-being and energy.

- Pleasure tools: for feeling good.

- Thinking tools: to stay in touch with reality.

- Social tools: to combat loneliness.

- Relaxation tools: to feel calm and confident.

These six tools comprise the Emotion Repair Toolbox for depression. As you can see, each tool is specifically designed to fix one of the reasons for on-going depression, just as real tools are designed for a particular job, for example a hammer is well designed for banging in a nail. Using just one of these tools may be enough to alleviate the sadness, but if you have a deep level of sadness, or the sadness has been around for a long time, you are likely to need several tools, possibly all six.

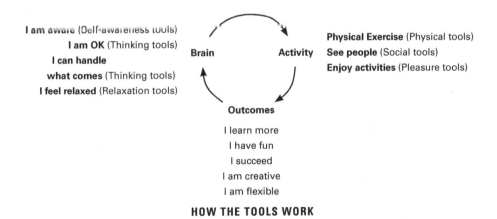

HOW THE TOOLS WORK

In the above diagram, you can see the way in which the six tools are used to combat depression, using the concept of the cycle of emotions discussed in stage 2 (see diagram on page 81). The self-awareness, thinking and relaxation tools have a positive repair effect on the brain. The physical, social and pleasure tools are constructive activities; they enable you to enjoy life more, achieve greater success, and be more creative, flexible and optimistic, both about yourself and the way in which you perceive life. Any or all of these tools, therefore, can help you reduce your level of depression.

During the next stages of the *Exploring Depression* programme we will be describing in detail each of the categories of emotion repair tools to assist you in creating your own, personal toolbox.

Self-awareness tools

You have already started to use a self-awareness tool, namely, the first activity in each of the stages that you have completed so far in this programme. Self-awareness is important for:

- Self-regulation: which enables you to understand what you are thinking and feeling so that you can perceive when you are feeling sad, and can then to do something constructive to repair your emotions.

- Planning a life that will suit you: from knowing how much sleep you need, to choosing a career, to how much socializing is optimal for you.

In the Emotion Repair Toolbox, a self-awareness tool could be represented by a compass. Self-awareness provides a compass to point the direction of travel in your journey into the future.

There is a large body of research that indicates that self-awareness helps us to become smarter, happier and calmer. You are beginning each stage of the programme by practising a self-awareness exercise before embarking on the designated activities. Try also to practise the self-awareness exercise on a daily basis, whether or not you are doing the programme that day. This will be one of your projects for the following stages of the programme.

In addition to your three- to five-minute self-awareness exercise, we encourage you to seek out a weekly class in either yoga, Qi Gong, Tai Chi, meditation or a martial art (particularly Tai Kwon Do). These are all effective self-awareness tools. If you are not sure which class to attend, conduct some research on the Internet to find a class that suits your personality and abilities.

Physical tools

Depression can have a 'paralyzing' effect, such that you may feel you do not want to do any physical activity. However, in the many Cognitive Behaviour Therapy programmes we have conducted to treat depression in our clients who have Asperger's syndrome, we have found that the majority of clients have reported that their most effective tool from the Emotion Repair Toolbox is actually daily physical exercise. Please note, this does not negate the value of the other tools, but instead provides compelling reasons to give physical tools a first priority.

Scientific studies by psychologists have established that energetic activity can significantly and powerfully improve a person's mood and clarity of thought. Thus, regular physical exercise can repair feelings of sadness and misery, as well as making you smarter and improving your concentration and memory. Psychologists are increasingly recommending that a regular exercise programme can, in many cases, be more effective than medication and psychotherapy in alleviating mild depression and anxiety.

Physical activity can also release endorphins in the brain, chemicals associated with feeling content. While we have recognized for generations the benefits of a healthy mind and body, unfortunately many of those who have Asperger's syndrome tend to consider themselves as clumsy and poorly coordinated, and may well have been teased at school for not being as agile or successful in team sports as peers. You may have a poor body image and believe that your body is not capable of energetic activity, and you may associate physical activity with discomfort.

For many of those with Asperger's syndrome, the most enjoyable activities are predominantly sedentary, such as time on the computer or watching television. Together with the lethargy that is so characteristic of depression, this lack of activity can result in weight gain and poor posture over a number of years. This in turn can inhibit motivation, or any thoughts of improving mood by energetic physical exercise.

However, a personal trainer may be able to assess your body type, level of fitness and personality, and design for you a tailored physical exercise programme, enabling you to achieve an increased level of fitness gradually. This may become one of your most important tools to achieve a sense of well-being, and an effective antidote to depression.

In the Emotion Repair Toolbox, a physical tool could be represented by a hammer.

Identifying your own physical tools

Think of your favourite physical activities that can:

- significantly improve your mood

- restore a sense of optimism

- energize you

- improve confidence in your abilities and self-image.

Some of these tools may be physical activities that you used to do but could enjoy doing again, activities you do now but could do more often, and new physical activities you would like to experience to see if they improve your mood and thinking.

The physical tools do not have to be team sports or ball games. They can include solitary sports such as cycling, attending a fitness centre, body building, martial arts, horse riding or swimming, or sessions with your personal trainer. You could even work alongside a friend or family member who enjoys engaging in regular physical exercise, or go for a run with your dog.

The physical tools can be divided into those that can be used at home and those used at school or work.

Make a list of the physical tools you can use at home, school or work.

HOME   **SCHOOL OR WORK**

_____   _____

_____   _____

_____   _____

_____   _____

_____   _____

_____   _____

_____   _____

Projects

3.1 Writing in your compliments diary

Remember to continue to give two compliments each day. Remember also any compliments that you receive. Record all these in your compliments diary.

3.2 Adding regular physical exercise to your weekly planner

On the next page is a weekly planner. Fill in, as you did in Stage 2, the activities in your life to which you are committed. Include, as before, a three- or five-minute self-awareness activity each day.

Think next about when would be a good time for one of the physical activities that you have chosen above for home, school or work. An essential component of this programme is to plan and engage in at least two 30-minute physical exercise sessions in the next week. Write them on the planner and ensure the planner is visible at home. Remember that if your energy levels are low and you lack motivation for a physical activity such as the scheduled visit to the gym, perhaps go for a walk or cycle to the shops instead. Some physical activity is better than none.

WEEKLY PLANNER STAGE 3		
Morning	**Afternoon**	**Evening**
Monday		
Tuesday		
Wednesday		
Thursday		
Friday		
Saturday		
Sunday		

Schedule: Physical activities (2 x 30-minute)
Self-awareness exercise (daily)

3.3 Recording your activity on your self-monitoring sheet

Use the self-monitoring sheet that follows for keeping a record of:

- when, and for how long, you did physical exercise

- the times that you practised the self-awareness exercise.

Try to do this at the end of each day. This will be reviewed in Stage 4.
Remember that 'cheating' with these charts is only cheating on yourself.

SELF-MONITORING STAGE 3	
Self-awareness exercise	Physical activity
Monday		
Tuesday		
Wednesday		
Thursday		
Friday		
Saturday		
Sunday		

STAGE 4

Art and Pleasure Tools

In Stage 4 you will:

★ understand the importance of expressing your emotions through art

★ discover pleasure tools in the Emotion Repair Toolbox

★ recognize the value of your special interest as a pleasure tool.

Activities and Projects for Stage 4

Activities

- Review of Stage 3.

- Self-awareness exercise.

- Using art to express feelings.

- Identifying pleasures in life.

Projects

4.1 Expressing sadness through art.

4.2 Identifying additional pleasures in life.

4.3 Writing your compliments diary.

4.4 Adding pleasurable activities to your weekly planner.

4.5 Recording your activities on your self-monitoring sheet, and rating your happiness.

Review of Stage 3

TOOLS FOR COMBATING DEPRESSION

In Stage 3 we discussed two tools for combating depression. What were they?

_____

_____

_____

_____

COMPLIMENTS

Have you received any compliments since you completed Stage 3? What were they?

_____

_____

_____

_____

FOLLOWING YOUR WEEKLY PLAN

One of your projects for Stage 3 was to follow a plan that you had made for incorporating two new tools (self-awareness and physical) into your daily life and complete a self-monitoring sheet to record when you remembered to do these two activities. Take another look at your self-monitoring sheet now and ask yourself these questions:

What helped you remember to use the tools?

_____

_____

_____

_____

What were the barriers to remembering or using the tools?

_____

_____

_____

_____

How did the tools affect your mood and abilities?

_____

_____

_____

_____

Self-awareness exercise

Before you begin this next stage of the programme, take three to five minutes to complete a self-awareness exercise of your choice (either *Bringing the Body into Awareness*, or *Bringing the Five Senses into Awareness* – see Appendix I or Appendix III). This will help you focus on the new material that follows.

Using art to express feelings

Human beings throughout the ages have used art (painting, sculpture, writing, photography, movie-making, music, etc.) to eloquently communicate and process their emotions and experiences. It is often the case that we suppress our negative emotions and experiences, because these can be difficult to talk about, and talking about them can sometimes make us feel worse, as we have to relive the thoughts and emotions. However, as discussed in Chapter 3, suppressing emotion is a coping mechanism that, while effective in the very short term, can in fact lead to deepening levels of depression and anxiety. If talking about your emotions is difficult or impossible, we highly recommend using art to express your sad feelings and experiences.

Consider the following questions:

What are some examples of art being successful in helping people to creatively express their sadness or anguish? Think of songs and music, paintings and photographs.

_____

_____

_____

_____

What are your favourite songs or images that eloquently and accurately express your sadness?

_____

_____

_____

_____

How can being creative or appreciative of the artistic expression of sadness alleviate your feelings of sadness?

_____

_____

_____

_____

Identifying pleasures in life

One very common experience of having sad feelings, or going through a depression, is that we no longer participate in pleasurable activities. When we feel down, pessimistic and lacking energy, we tend to forget about the activities that used to bring us pleasure, and we don't have the energy to engage in them, or the belief that they could make us feel happy again. However, if you think about it logically, it would make sense that doing something you have enjoyed in the past could possibly help you to feel better.

What are your pleasures in life? What activities, experiences, thoughts, memories, people (and animals), and dreams of the future, or memories of the past, create within you a feeling of well-being and optimism? In the following activity, consider both past and current pleasures, and list as many as you can, as indicated.

ACTIVITIES

Past	Present
_____	_____
_____	_____
_____	_____
_____	_____
_____	_____
_____	_____

EXPERIENCES

Past	Present
_____	_____
_____	_____
_____	_____
_____	_____
_____	_____

THOUGHTS

Past	Present
_____	_____
_____	_____
_____	_____
_____	_____
_____	_____

MEMORIES

Past   *Present*

_____   _____

_____   _____

_____   _____

_____   _____

_____   _____

_____   _____

PEOPLE AND ANIMALS

Past   *Present*

_____   _____

_____   _____

_____   _____

_____   _____

_____   _____

_____   _____

DREAMS OF THE FUTURE

Past   *Present*

_____   _____

_____   _____

_____   _____

_____   _____

_____   _____

The value of a special interest

You may have a special interest – that is, a topic or activity that you really enjoy. You may have a natural ability in an area such as music, mathematics, fine art, or remembering facts and information, or have a collection of objects that give you pleasure, or be highly practised and have a reputation in a specific computer game. Lots of practice and time devoted to the interest may lead to recognized and appreciated success and intense personal enjoyment when engaged in this special topic.

The degree of enjoyment you experience when engaged in your special interest may be far superior to any of the other pleasures in your life.

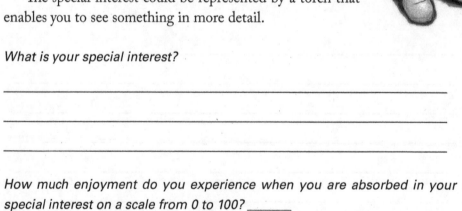

Intense happiness, success and enjoyment are powerful antidotes to feeling sad. Nick Dubin, an adult author with Asperger's syndrome, has written in his excellent book on depression, 'I have never met anyone with Asperger's syndrome who was depressed when they were involved with a special interest.'[6]

Your special interest can restore energy and strengthen self-esteem, as well as act as a thought blocker to anxious or sad thoughts.

Thus, your special interest, because of the pleasure it provides you, can be a very useful tool in the Emotion Repair Toolbox.

Be aware, however, that it can be so enjoyable that you may be criticized by others for spending too much time engaged it. When that occurs, you will need alternative tools in your toolbox.

The special interest could be represented by a torch that enables you to see something in more detail.

What is your special interest?

_____

_____

_____

How much enjoyment do you experience when you are absorbed in your special interest on a scale from 0 to 100? _____

6   Dubin, N. (2014) *The Autism Spectrum and Depression*. London: Jessica Kingsley Publishers.

Projects

4.1 Expressing sadness through art

It can be difficult to express feelings in face-to-face conversation, and some people find a better way to do this is through engaging in various forms of artistic expression. The aim of this project is for you to either find an example of existing art, or create something of your own, that helps you express your feelings of sadness. Here are some suggestions to help:

- find a section of music or a song

- find a photograph or a painting

- find part of a movie

- find a poem or a short story

- find a sculpture

- write a song or piece of music

- take a photograph

- create a video

- write a poem or a short story

- create a sculpture or collage.

Either by yourself or with someone who is important in your life, spend some time looking at, reading, listening to, and admiring the work of art that you have chosen to accurately and eloquently express your feelings. Allow yourself to experience any sadness that arises as a result of this activity. Notice where you feel your sadness in your body. For some, it is in their throat, for others, in the region of their chest; still others locate their sadness in their stomach, or find tears cascading down their cheeks. There is no right or wrong in this exercise: it simply allows you to be in touch with how your body reacts to or expresses sadness.

Next, rate your sadness, using a scale of 0–100 (see the Sadness Thermometer on page 79).

My level of sadness _____

It may be difficult to talk about this, and to share the expression and emotion with someone you care about. However, we highly recommend that you do take this step. Sometimes, it is difficult to talk things over with someone such as partner, parent or friend. If this is the case for you, consider that it may be easier to see someone independent of your life, for example, a psychologist with experience in Asperger's syndrome and depression. If there is no such person near where you live, scan your life to see if there is someone from the past, or a member of your extended family with whom you may be able to share the work of art.

4.2 Identifying additional pleasures in life

Talk with the person providing support and guidance as you complete the programme about the pleasures you have in life, and together add to the list you created earlier (see pages 114–115). Remember, these thoughts and experiences can act as antidotes to feeling sad or depressed, and will be further explored during the next stage of the programme.

4.3 Writing in your compliments diary

Continue to give two compliments a day, and record in your compliments diary those that you have received.

4.4 Adding pleasurable activities to your weekly planner

There are now three activities to schedule in to your weekly plan, in addition to your regular commitments and chores. This time you will be increasing the number of physical activities from two to three (or four, if you can manage it) times in the week. You will continue to include your self-awareness exercise each day, at a time that suits you best; and now, in addition, you will add one pleasurable activity every day. Take these from the list of activities you identified earlier as helpful to you (see pages 114–115).

Add to the weekly planner:

- physical activities (3–4 times)

- self-awareness exercise (daily)

- pleasurable activities (daily).

WEEKLY PLANNER STAGE 4		
Morning	Afternoon	Evening
Monday		
Tuesday		
Wednesday		
Thursday		
Friday		
Saturday		
Sunday		

Schedule: Physical activities (3–4)
Self-awareness exercise (daily)
Pleasurable activities (daily)

4.5 Recording your activities on your self-monitoring sheet, and rating your happiness

At this stage, use the self-monitoring sheet provided to record:

- when, and for how long, you did a physical exercise (3–4 times a week)

- the times you practised the self-awareness exercise (daily)

- when you included some form of pleasurable activity (daily)

- how you felt (using a happiness scale 0–100) *before* and *after* each of the exercises and activities.

SELF-MONITORING STAGE 4

| | Self-awareness exercise 1 | Physical activity 2 | Pleasurable activity 3 | Rating (0–100) | | | | | | |
| | | | | Before | | | After | | |
				1	2	3	1	2	3
Monday									
Tuesday									
Wednesday									
Thursday									
Friday									
Saturday									
Sunday									

Making changes: Keeping up the momentum

Part of being human is that, even with the best of intentions and the highest levels of motivation, we set ourselves goals and then do not take action. There can be a tendency for distractions and procrastination. If at this stage in the programme you are finding that you are experiencing difficulty in completing the projects (separately to reading the book) you are not alone.

If you are completing this programme with the guidance of someone that you know, we highly recommend discussing with that person any difficulties that you are having in completing the projects, and your motivation.

You may find it helpful to consider the following suggestions to help you stay positive and focused:

- Start noticing your successes, rather than dwelling on a perceived sense of failure.

- Take note of any progress that you make within this programme, no matter how small you tell yourself that is.

- Remind yourself on a daily basis that taking steps toward change is difficult and challenging, and that some people may consider giving up at this stage.

- Tell yourself that you resolve to not be one of those people.

- Remind yourself that while there is pain in change, there is even more pain in staying depressed, and, as a result, living a life that makes you feel even more depressed.

- Start to see the pain involved in making changes as being the pain involved in growing as a person.

- Commit to the pathway of growing as a person.

- Do what you need to do to be your own life coach, for example:

  ○ list all the benefits that you can see will come from living your life as a non-depressed person

  ○ pin your list up on the fridge or somewhere you will easily see it

  ○ use an affirmation that feels good to you, every single day (see below).

Positive affirmations

These are some examples of affirmations that have helped many people with anxiety and depression:

- I can make the changes I want to in my life.

- I am powerful in my own life.

- I love myself unconditionally.

- I am STRONG!

- I allow only healthy and loving relationships into my life.

- Life wants the best for me. I am OK with where I am right now.

- I am connected and comfortable in all environments, with all people.

- I find and enjoy the simple pleasures life is offering right now.

- How I feel matters, therefore I concentrate on aspects of life that make me feel good.

- My challenges bring me better opportunities.

- My mood creates a physiological response in my body. I am peaceful and positive.

- I am in control of my thoughts and my life.

- I love myself and who I am.[7]

---

7   See www.powerofpositivity.com

Thinking Tools (Part 1)

In Stage 5, you will:

★ explore the value of five thinking tools in the Emotion Repair Toolbox.

Activities and Projects for Stage 5

Activities

- Review of Stage 4.
- Self-awareness exercise.
- Giving compliments to yourself.
- Appreciating enjoyable aspects of your life.
- Imagining what your hero would do.
- Creating a pleasures diary.
- Applying a reality check.

Projects

5.1 Writing in your compliments diary.

5.2 Recognizing and measuring happiness and sadness.

5.3 Filling in your weekly planner.

5.4 Self-monitoring.

Review of Stage 4

Why is it important to schedule pleasurable activities into your week?

_____

_____

_____

_____

Why is it important to schedule a wide range of pleasurable experiences other than your special interest during your week?

_____

_____

_____

_____

ADDING NEW TOOLS TO YOUR WEEKLY PLAN

You have been encouraged to follow a plan that incorporates new emotion repair tools into your life, namely, two extra physical activities and a daily pleasurable activity. You have also completed a self-monitoring sheet to record when you remembered to do these activities, and how you felt before and after doing them. Look at your self-monitoring sheet now and answer the following questions:

What helped you to remember to use the tools?

_____

_____

_____

_____

What were the barriers to remembering or using the tools?

_____

_____

_____

_____

How could you overcome some of those barriers?

_____

_____

_____

_____

How did you feel before and after your physical exercise?

_____

_____

_____

_____

EXPRESSING SADNESS THROUGH ART

You selected examples of expressions of art or music that helped you describe your feelings of sadness. Look at, or listen to, this selection again, and reflect on how you felt when you shared this art or music with someone else:

_____

_____

_____

_____

ADDITIONAL PLEASURES IN LIFE

You were asked to discuss with your family members or friends, any other pleasurable activities that you could think of to add to your list of pleasures, past and present. Did you and they come up with any extra ideas? What were they?

_____

_____

_____

_____

COMPLIMENTS

Did you remember to give two compliments each day, and to write in your compliments diary any that you received? What were some of the compliments that you gave or received during Stage 4?

_____

_____

_____

_____

Self-awareness exercise

Complete a three- or five-minute self-awareness exercise to refresh you and prepare your mind for the information and activities in Stage 5 (see Appendix I or Appendix III).

Thinking tools

Thinking tools change perception, knowledge, beliefs and reactions. Thinking tools use intellectual strength to analyze, evaluate and repair feelings of sadness.

They can be conceptualized as a repair manual.

Thinking tools for Stage 5 include:

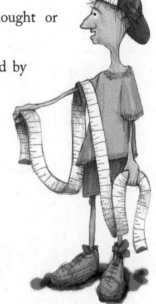

- giving yourself a compliment: change a negative self-perception that creates pessimism about your abilities or future to a positive one that creates optimism and self-worth

- noticing something in your environment or life that you appreciate

- imagining what your hero would do in your situation

- creating a pleasures diary that records in words or photographs any pleasures you experience, providing examples of what makes life worthwhile

- applying a reality check: is the event, thought or comment actually as serious as you believe?

Thinking tools could also, therefore, be represented by a tape measure that measures the real significance of an event or the dimensions of your qualities, achievements and pleasures.

In the following sections, you will be guided through the application of each of these thinking tools in a structured way.

Giving compliments to yourself

Choose four situations that make you feel sad. What compliment could you give yourself as an antidote to poisonous thoughts and feelings that make you feel sad? For example, you could think that you are a loser, but you are actually a winner when you play Minecraft; or you might think, 'everyone hates me', but the antidote could be, 'my mother/partner loves me and is a good judge of character.' It is also worth bearing in mind that one of the characteristics of increasing maturity is that as you get older, you genuinely care less what people think of you.

The compliment may be one that you create for yourself or one that you have received from someone else – perhaps one that you have recorded in your compliments diary.

Situation 1:

_____

_____

Compliment:

_____

_____

Situation 2:

_____

_____

Compliment:

_____

_____

Situation 3:

_____

_____

Compliment:

_____

_____

Situation 4:

_____

_____

Compliment:

_____

_____

Appreciating enjoyable aspects of your life

What can you see, hear, smell or touch in the room where you are at the moment that makes you feel good?

_____

_____

_____

_____

What quality in yourself do you most admire?

_____

_____

_____

_____

What achievement are you most proud of?

_____

_____

_____

_____

What is one of the pleasures in your life at the moment?

_____

_____

_____

_____

Thinking about what you enjoy and look forward to can be an antidote to sad or pessimistic thoughts. What are the aspects of your life that you enjoy or are grateful for? These could include aspects of yourself (characteristics, talents, health, etc.), someone in your life, or your pet, or pastimes or interests that you enjoy.

_____

_____

_____

_____

_____

Imagining what your hero would do

There may be someone, real or fictitious, whom you consider to be your hero. This might be someone in literature or films, someone in public life, past or present, or even a family member or friend. You may admire this person's qualities, and the way he or she approaches life, dealing with problems and obstacles as they arise. Another thinking tool is to imagine what this 'hero' would do in a particular situation. Please be careful in choosing your hero. Some of the violent justice and retribution dispensed by 'superheroes' in films and computer games is neither realistic nor advisable.

Who is your hero?

_____

_____

What qualities does he or she have that you admire?

_____

_____

_____

_____

Imagine what your hero would do or say in the four situations that make you feel sad that you described previously (see pages 129–130). How could you adopt their qualities and abilities to not feel sad?

Situation 1: You could:

_____

_____

_____

_____

Situation 2: You could:

_____

_____

_____

_____

Situation 3: You could:

_____

_____

_____

_____

Situation 4: You could:

_____

_____

_____

_____

Creating a pleasures diary

Create a diary in which you record moments of happiness, success or enjoyment. Whenever you experience something that you would like to recall as an antidote to feelings of sadness, and to encourage optimism for the future, record it in your pleasures diary. You can then look at it later to remind you that life has, and will continue to have, pleasurable moments.

These moments can be minor events or experiences, which may in fact not stand out in the moment – it can be watching a good movie, or doing something kind for someone else, or giving them a compliment. It can be completing your physical exercise for the day. Anything you can think of to say, 'I did this.'

The record could be text, a photograph or a memento, such as a cinema ticket, that helps you re-connect with moments of happiness.

Applying a reality check

Consider this situation:

> You are waiting at the movie theatre for your friend to arrive. The movie starts at 6.30 p.m. and you had arranged to meet at 6 p.m. to buy the tickets, a drink and something to eat. It is now 6.25 p.m. and there is no sign of your friend.

Person A starts to think: 'What did I do wrong last time I spoke to my friend? He seemed fine and agreed to go to the pictures, but now he has not turned up. I just know he no longer likes me. Just like all the other times I have tried to make a friend. I will never make a friend. I am hopeless and unlikeable. There is just something terribly wrong with me.'

How is Person A feeling?

_____

_____

_____

_____

Why do you think he feels this way?

_____

_____

_____

_____

What is the evidence for the thought, 'I am hopeless and unlikeable'?

_____

_____

_____

_____

Person B is in the same situation. He starts to think: 'I do hope that something bad hasn't happened to my friend. He is usually very reliable. It is unusual for him to be 10 minutes late. The bus he catches may have been held up. The traffic was very bad getting here.'

How is Person B feeling?

_____

_____

_____

_____

Why do you think he feels this way?

_____

_____

_____

_____

What is the difference between Person B's thinking style, compared to that of Person A?

_____

_____

_____

_____

Do you tend to think like Person A? If so, in what ways?

_____

_____

_____

_____

How could you think more like Person B?

_____

_____

_____

_____

Describe a situation that you have experienced over the last few weeks where your thinking may have been pessimistic and self-critical, like Person A:

_____

_____

_____

_____

How could you change your perception of the situation and your thinking, so that they are based on a more realistic and objective analysis of the situation?

_____

_____

_____

_____

(If you are unsure how to change your thoughts about the situation, and not jump to conclusions, ask a family member or friend or the person giving you guidance for this programme for their interpretation of the situation.)

_____

_____

_____

_____

Consider four more situations that have occurred recently that you could re-examine and to which you could apply an alternative thinking style.

Situation 1:

_____

_____

You could:

_____

_____

_____

Situation 2:

_____

_____

You could:

_____

_____

_____

Situation 3:

_____

_____

You could:

_____

_____

_____

Situation 4:

_____

_____

You could:

_____

_____

_____

Projects

5.1 Writing in your compliments diary

Continue to record compliments that you have given and received.

5.2 Recognizing and measuring happiness and sadness

Between now and starting Stage 6, choose a time when you feel particularly happy or have a happy thought, and record this below.

What happened?

_____

_____

_____

_____

What were your happy thoughts?

_____

_____

_____

_____

How happy were you on a scale from 0 to 100 where 0 is 'neutral' and 100 is 'ecstatic'?

    Your score _____

Next, choose a time when you feel sad or have a sad thought, and record this below.

What happened?

_____

_____

_____

_____

What were your sad thoughts?

_____

_____

_____

_____

How sad were you on a scale from 0 to 100, where 0 is 'neutral' and 100 is 'suicidal'?

Your score _____

These two situations and your thoughts will be explored in the next stage of the programme.

5.3 Filling in your weekly planner

As in Stage 4, fill in your weekly planner, including your regular chores and commitments. Also include:

- physical activities (3–4 times)
- self-awareness exercise (daily)
- pleasurable activities (daily).

WEEKLY PLANNER STAGE 5		
Morning	**Afternoon**	**Evening**
Monday			
Tuesday			
Wednesday			
Thursday			
Friday			
Saturday			
Sunday			

Schedule: Physical activities (3–4)

Self-awareness exercise (daily)

Pleasurable activities (daily)

5.4 Self-monitoring

PHYSICAL ACTIVITIES, SELF-AWARENESS EXERCISE AND PLEASURABLE ACTIVITIES

Use the self-monitoring sheet that follows to record, as you have previously, when you complete your three or four sessions of physical activity, your daily self-awareness exercise and your daily pleasurable activities.

Once again, there is space for rating on your happiness scale (0–100) how you felt before and after each of these activities.

THINKING TOOLS

Now, use the self-monitoring sheet to record your use of thinking tools. There may be times during the coming week when your thoughts are overly negative, pessimistic or catastrophic. Use one (or more) of the five thinking tools to change your thoughts. Remember, the five thinking tools are:

- giving yourself a compliment, not a criticism

- appreciating an enjoyable aspect of your life to cheer yourself up

- imagining what your hero would do in that situation and consider that, should that situation happen again, you can 'act' as your hero

- creating and looking at your pleasures diary to help change your thoughts from pessimistic to optimistic

- applying a reality check: be a scientist or detective, and check the actual evidence for a particular thought.

Record which thinking tool or tools you used, and rate your level of happiness before and after using the tool.

SELF-MONITORING STAGE 5

	Self-awareness exercise 1	Physical activity 2	Pleasurable activity 3	Thinking tools 4	Rating (0–100)							
					Before				After			
					1	2	3	4	1	2	3	4
Monday												
Tuesday												
Wednesday												
Thursday												
Friday												
Saturday												
Sunday												

Thinking Tools (Part 2) and Social Tools

In Stage 6, you will:

★ learn more about thinking tools in the Emotion Repair Toolbox

★ explore social tools in the Emotion Repair Toolbox.

Activities and Projects for Stage 6

Activities

- Review of Stage 5.

- Self-awareness exercise.

- Challenging and changing your thoughts.

Projects

6.1 Writing in your compliments diary.

6.2 Adding a social activity to your weekly planner.

6.3 Self-monitoring.

6.4 Thinking activity: Challenging distortions in thinking.

Review of Stage 5

How can changing your thinking change your feelings?

_____

_____

_____

_____

What was one of the compliments you gave yourself in Stage 5 (see pages 129–130)?

_____

_____

_____

_____

How could your hero model how to be positive and cope with adversity?

_____

_____

_____

CONTINUING SELF-AWARENESS, PHYSICAL AND PLEASURABLE ACTIVITIES IN YOUR WEEKLY PLAN

You have continued to follow a weekly plan that incorporates a daily self-awareness activity, three to four physical activities and a daily pleasurable activity. You have recorded on your self-monitoring sheet when you remembered to do these activities in the last week, as well as recording how you felt after each of them. Have a look at the self-monitoring sheet now and consider these questions:

What helped you to remember to use the tools?

_____

_____

_____

_____

What were the barriers to remembering or using the tools?

_____

_____

_____

_____

What could you do to overcome these barriers?

_____

_____

_____

_____

How did you feel before and after your physical exercise?

_____

_____

_____

_____

Which pleasurable activities did you schedule?

1. _____

_____

2. _____

_____

How did these pleasurable activities go?

1. _____

_____

2. _____

_____

EXPLORING DEPRESSION, AND BEATING THE BLUES

RECOGNIZING AND MEASURING HAPPINESS AND SADNESS

What were some examples of your sad thoughts?

_____

_____

_____

_____

What were some examples of your happy thoughts?

_____

_____

_____

_____

What is the connection between your thinking and how you felt?

_____

_____

_____

_____

Self-awareness exercise

Before commencing Stage 6 activities, take three to five minutes to complete your favourite self-awareness exercise now (*Bringing the Body into Awareness* or *Bringing the Five Senses into Awareness* – see Appendix I or Appendix III). Pausing to do this will clear your mind from any previous activities, allowing you to process the new information more effortlessly and efficiently.

Thinking tools (Part 2)
Challenging and changing your thoughts

Think again about the sad thoughts you identified in Project 5.2. Ask yourself:

What was the evidence to confirm your sad thoughts?

_____

_____

_____

_____

What could be alternative objective, realistic or even optimistic thoughts in that situation? Remember, being optimistic is not being delusionally happy. It is thinking, 'I am not going to let this get me down, I will think positive thoughts.'

Objective and realistic thoughts:

_____

_____

_____

_____

Optimistic and positive thoughts:

_____

_____

_____

_____

Perception is everything

You learned in Stage 5 that although we cannot change some situations, we do have some control over how we feel and react to them, and through our thoughts and actions we can repair our feelings of sadness and depression. In other words, the way we think about a situation determines in large part how we feel about that situation. We have a choice. Unfortunately, when we are tired, anxious, stressed or depressed, our automatic or default thinking style tends to be pessimistic; thus, our thoughts can actually keep us depressed and stressed if we let them. The trick is to recognize this pattern of thinking and not believe our first, or pessimistic, thought.

Common distortions in thinking in depression

Professor Aaron Beck, now considered the 'father' of Cognitive Behaviour Therapy, was the first to identify the following common distortions in thinking that occur when we are depressed. We include these here because there is now considerable evidence, as reviewed in Chapter 4, that identifying and challenging our negative thoughts can be a useful tool in our Emotion Repair Toolbox for dealing with strong emotions as they arise.

Please note, often we need to consider our thinking *after* the event, since at the time we may be too emotional to think logically and clearly enough to identify any thinking distortion. However, the more often we reflect on our habitual ways of thinking, the more quickly we learn to challenge our thinking distortions and stop believing the error messages. The result is that we experience increased feelings of well-being and calm.

You may be able to see here how important the self-awareness exercises that you have been practising throughout the programme become. Without self-awareness, these unhelpful thinking patterns happen quite automatically, and the resulting rush of negative emotion can be very difficult to manage.

Here are the most common thinking distortions:

- *Black-and-white thinking*: You think things are always one way or the other, for example 'I can never do anything right' or 'It will never work, I will always be lonely.'

- *Overgeneralization*: Just because one thing goes wrong, you think everything will go wrong: 'It is the eternal pattern of my life.'

- *Magical thinking*: You think you will have a bad day or something bad will happen based on the occurrence of something else completely unrelated – a superstitious reaction, for example 'I saw five yellow cars this morning, yellow cars are bad luck, so today will be a bad day' or 'I seem to have been cursed all my life.'

- *Mental filter*: You see the world through a filter that effectively prevents any positive thoughts or events entering your mind.

- *Disqualifying the positive*: If something good happens you dismiss it as being irrelevant or unique and never to be repeated: 'They didn't really mean it'; or to be rejected because it is not consistent with your pessimistic beliefs about yourself.

- *Jumping to conclusions*: You decide that you know what someone is thinking or feeling and what will happen in the future, even though you can't read someone else's mind or tell the future. These are:

  ○ mind reading

  ○ fortune (or disaster) foretelling.

- *Magnification and minimization*: You magnify the problem so that is all you see, and minimize the positive. This distortion is:

  ○ catastrophizing (can be a characteristic of Asperger's syndrome).

- *Emotional reasoning*: You think because you feel it, it must be true.

- *'Should' statements*: Your thoughts reflect rigid rules about how you or others 'should' behave, such as, 'I should have known better' or 'I should have read the signals.'

- *Labelling and mislabelling*: You rely on naming yourself, others or events, and therefore miss out on a deeper or more accurate understanding of yourself, others or events, for example 'I am a loser', 'I am a natural victim', or 'That was a disaster.'

- *Personalization*: You think, 'It was all my fault', even when you did not have control over everything that happened.

Do you recognize any of these patterns of thinking in yourself?

Black-and-white thinking ____

Overgeneralization ____

Magical thinking ____

Mental filter ____

Disqualifying the positive ____

Jumping to conclusions ____

Magnification and minimization ____

Emotional reasoning ____

'Should' statements ____

Labelling and mislabelling ____

Personalization ____

Ways to challenge the distortions in thinking
Black-and-white thinking
Things are rarely black and white; can you see the shades of grey in the situation?

Instead of 'always' insert the word 'sometimes'.

Look for the exception in what you are thinking.

Thinking distortion: There is no point trying, I always fail.

Realistic thinking: I can learn from my mistakes. I can ask for help. If I ask for help, people will think I am constructively trying to solve the problem and that I am a friendly and wise person. There are many ways to solve the problem. If I keep trying, it is likely I will soon succeed.

Overgeneralization
Get back to the specifics. Think only about this moment, this time, this situation.

Thinking distortion: Grace did not call back, even though she said she would. I will never be able to make a good friend.

Realistic thinking: Grace may have forgotten that she said she would call as she is incredibly busy at the moment. The battery of her mobile/cell phone may be dead. If Grace does not want to be friends, there are many other people in the world. I will find others who may become good friends.

Magical thinking

Remind yourself that the concepts you are linking are totally unrelated. Just because one thing happened does not mean another thing will happen. Check if you are creating faulty logic.

Thinking distortion: If I arrange all the cutlery in the cutlery drawer perfectly, today will go well.

Realistic thinking: I enjoy arranging all the cutlery in the cutlery drawer. Today will go well if I stay focused on what is happening in the moment and try to keep a positive attitude. Arranging the cutlery could not influence the actual events that I experience, but could affect how I perceive the events of the day.

Mental filter

Are you looking at the total situation, or focusing only on a few details? Those who have Asperger's syndrome tend to over-focus on details, especially errors. Mentally, take at least one step back and rethink the situation. Try to see what you are missing; look for the 'big picture', the overall effect. Ask someone else for their perspective if you cannot see it. There is always more information out there, and always many more perspectives than just one.

Thinking distortion: I always see the rain. I never feel the sunshine. I am saturated and drowning with problems and mistakes.

Realistic thinking: A few things in my day today were difficult for me to deal with. However, there were some positive events. As a result of so many genuine difficulties, I feel tired and negative. I will look after myself tonight, make sure I have a healthy dinner and a good sleep, and tomorrow when I feel rested and better, I can think about the good moments in the day and what I have learned.

Disqualifying the positive

The good things that are happening are just as relevant and important as the bad things that are happening. Start to trust that good things will happen to you, as well as bad things.

Thinking distortion: Only bad things ever happen to me. When people say something nice to me, they do it out of pity. The best event of my day happened because of luck, so it doesn't mean anything.

Realistic thinking: Both good and bad things happen to me. I will make an effort to notice when good things are happening. I will amplify and accept these things into my life. I will get events into perspective and in balance.

Jumping to conclusions
No one knows the future. We cannot read minds. Start to accept that there will be uncertainty in life, and you will not always know what will lie ahead; this can be a good thing.

Thinking distortion: This friendship will end badly, they always do.

Realistic thinking: I cannot predict the future. If I stay present to what is happening and keep a positive attitude, I can increase the chance of things working out well in this friendship, and I can learn from this experience to help with future friendships and relationships.

Magnification and minimization
Figuratively speaking, take out the mirror, not the magnifying glass, and don't reverse the telescope. Look at the situation, or yourself, realistically rather than focusing only on what is wrong.

Thinking distortion: I am a failure.

Realistic thinking: I made a mistake today, but I can learn from my mistake and next time I may be able to achieve success. Learning from mistakes makes me smarter and wiser.

Emotional reasoning
Feeling or thinking that something is true does not automatically make it true.

Thinking distortion: I will always feel sad.

Realistic thinking: Just because I feel strongly that I will always feel sad does not mean it is true. I can take steps, like the ones in this programme, to overcome my sadness and start to feel pleasure and happiness again, and enjoy being me.

'Should' statements

Having high personal expectations and seeking perfection can make it harder to accept your mistakes.

Thinking distortion: I should be perfect and I should never make a mistake.

Realistic thinking: No one is perfect and everyone makes mistakes. I don't like making mistakes but they are inevitable. I will try to stay calm so that I can stay smart and learn from this mistake.

Labelling and mislabelling

No person or situation can be solely defined by one label. Practising this way of thinking will seriously limit your understanding of a situation and your ability to be flexible in your perception and response.

Thinking distortion: I am stupid.

Realistic thinking: Stupid is a negative label that will just make me feel bad. We can all do and say things that sometimes seem stupid, but this does not mean that we are stupid.

Personalization

Take a step back and view the situation objectively. Consider which parts of the situation you had control of or were responsible for, and which parts you didn't. Remember that you can never control someone else's behaviour or reaction to you, but you can control your own reaction

Thinking distortion: I did not get that job because I am a failure.

Realistic thinking: I do not know why I did not get that job. There could be a number of reasons. Maybe there were a lot of applicants, and the best applicant had more experience than I have. Maybe I did not come across well for the job interview. I can learn some skills to prepare well for future job interviews, to potentially make it a success next time. I will not let this get me down.

Now that you have absorbed the challenges (in the form of realistic thinking) to the most common examples of distorted and dysfunctional thinking, are there any that stand out as being particularly relevant and important for you? List them below:

_____

_____

_____

_____

_____

Learning how to apply social tools

It is now time to introduce another category of tool in your personal Emotion Repair Toolbox, and that is social tools.

Social tools could be represented by a sponge that 'cleanses' the feeling.

People (and animals) in your life

There are several social tools, one of the most effective of which is being with people who can help you repair feelings of sadness, in several ways: by being supportive; believing in your qualities; validating your feelings; cheering you up; putting an event in perspective; correcting any distortions in thinking; and 'soaking up' your despair.

There is wisdom in the phrase, 'A problem shared is a problem halved.' And it is logical to employ a number of different perspectives, strategies and styles of thinking when looking at a situation. In this way, you will have access to much more knowledge and wisdom. When you ask for someone else's opinion or advice, you immediately double the brainpower applied to the problem. Even if you do not agree with everything they say, allow yourself to be open to the possibility that there may be an alternative way to solve the problem, and a different perception of the situation or your abilities.

When adding a person to your social tool box, ensure that he or she is a good listener, non-judgemental, validates your feelings and gives emotional and practical support, reassurance and compliments, not criticism or expressions of disappointment.

The emotional repair may not be via a face-to-face conversation, but involve communication through the Internet, text or telephone.

Another special and powerful social tool is for you to engage in helping someone else in an act of kindness or generosity. Being needed and valued is a very effective emotional repair mechanism for feelings of low self-worth.

Yet another social tool can be the presence of an animal in your life, perhaps your pet, who may be your 'best friend'.

Who could you include in the social tools section of your Emotion Repair Toolbox?

At home:

_____

_____

Outside home, for example work or school:

_____

_____

How could that person (or animal) help?

At home:

_____

_____

Outside home, for example work or school:

_____

_____

Increasing social activities

It is important to have enjoyable social contact: it is a very fundamental human need. There are several ways to do this. You could begin by considering how you may be able to connect to people who also have Asperger's syndrome. This may be through your local Asperger's support group, or through a website. We include a list of potential websites you can contact at the end of the book.

If you would like to increase your social contacts, but not necessarily with people who have Asperger's syndrome, consider your own interests and hobbies as a starting point. Could you join an interest group? There are many groups for all sorts of interests and activities, such as chess, role playing games, anime, train spotting, photography, bushwalking, dog training, horse riding, science, geology, learning a new language, dance, yoga, meditation, church, gardening, and so on. If you cannot find the right group to join, maybe consider enrolling in a course to learn more about your interest. We often find that like minds attract. You may find there are others in your interest or study group who think like you, or have similar interests. Seeing each other outside the group is a good way to build friendships. If you are interested in keeping in touch with other group members, you can swap contact details, and enjoy friendship via social media or phone, as well as conversations in the group itself.

Many people who have Asperger's syndrome are avoidant of social contact because of past bad experiences, such as being rejected, teased, humiliated or bullied. However, even if this is the case for you, please consider that having bad experiences in the past *does not* predict all your future experience. Each day is new, literally. Also, you do not need to find a large group of friends to be happy, but all of us need at least one person who likes who we are, just as we are. This is a very basic human need. Focus on finding just one friend.

Without this social contact, depression is, unfortunately, a likely outcome. Remember, also, just as you do not need a large group of friends, you do not need a large number of social activities on your calendar. We recommend trialling just one social activity per week. But if this is too much, cut it back. If it is not enough, increase.

Projects

6.1 Writing in your compliments diary

Continue to record compliments that you have given and received.

6.2 Adding a social activity to your weekly planner

As well as your regular appointments and commitments, there are four types of activities to schedule for Stage 6. There are the three activities that you have already been scheduling:

- physical activities (3–4 times)

- self-awareness exercises (daily)

- pleasurable activities (daily).

Now, at Stage 6, you will include one social activity per week. Think about a time in the coming week that you can schedule something social, for example, discovering a local interest group that appeals to you and attending a meeting; emailing an old friend; talking to someone on the telephone; going to the movies with someone you like, etc.

EXPLORING DEPRESSION, AND BEATING THE BLUES

WEEKLY PLANNER STAGE 6		
	Morning	Afternoon	Evening
Monday			
Tuesday			
Wednesday			
Thursday			
Friday			
Saturday			
Sunday			

Schedule: Physical activities (3–4)

Self-awareness exercise (daily)

Pleasurable activities (daily)

Social activity (1)

6.3 Self-monitoring

Use the self-monitoring sheet that follows to record, as you have previously, when you complete your daily self-awareness exercise and physical activities, and your pleasurable activities and social activities. There is, as before, space for rating how you felt before and after each activity, using a happiness scale from 0 to 100.

SELF-MONITORING SHEET STAGE 6

	Self-awareness exercise 1	Physical activity 2	Pleasurable activity 3	Social activity 4	Rating (0–100) Before				After			
					1	2	3	4	1	2	3	4
Monday												
Tuesday												
Wednesday												
Thursday												
Friday												
Saturday												
Sunday												

6.4 Thinking activity: Challenging distortions in thinking

Read through the following thinking activity based on an imaginary event. This will prepare you for the activities in Stage 7.

A friend tells you that he does not want to hang around with you anymore because you are not 'cool'.

1. List the emotions you feel. Rate the intensity of each of these emotions, on a scale of 0 to 10 (10 being the most intense), for example devastated 9/10; confused 7/10, etc.

_____   _____

_____   _____

_____   _____

_____   _____

_____   _____

_____   _____

2. Circle any of the following thoughts that may have come along with the emotion you have just described. Add your own if you have one.

a) I must be 'uncool' and boring.

b) Maybe other people think I am not 'cool'.

c) I am not very likeable.

d) I will never make another friend and will be friendless forever.

e) _____

_____

3. Recognize the thinking distortions for each of the thoughts in Question 2. Identify the distortion in your additional thought:

    a) mislabelling and magnification

    b) mind-reading

    c) mislabelling and overgeneralization

    d) fortune-telling and catastrophizing

    e) _____

4. Write down a rational response to the thought. These are examples of rational responses, including responses to each of the suggested thoughts in Question 2:

    a) Just because one person thinks I am not 'cool' doesn't mean that everyone will. He may have reasons for saying that that are nothing to do with me, and that I do not know about.

    b) Other people may think I am not 'cool', but that is okay, I don't have to be wildly interesting and exciting to everyone. There will be people who think I am interesting and perhaps 'cool' in a different way.

    c) Just because one person says that I am not 'cool', it does not mean that I am unlikeable. Being uncool may not mean unlikeable, and even if it does, it is still only one person saying it. Other people will find me likeable. There is a lot of variety in the world.

    d) Just because one friendship has come to an end does not mean that there will never be another friendship. Friendships break up all the time. Friendships often have a 'use by' date. I have made friends with other people, and will continue to do so.

    e) Do I want someone like that to like me anyway?

    f) The person who made the comment has moved on and probably has no idea of the hurt caused.

    g) _____

_____

5. *Are there any other rational responses to each thought?*

a) _____

_____

b) _____

_____

c) _____

_____

d) _____

_____

e) _____

_____

6. *Think about the event again, then read your rational responses. List the emotions you feel now. As you did in Question 1, rate each of these emotions on a scale of 0 to 10. Compare your original thoughts and ratings with your new thoughts and ratings, now that you have challenged the distortions in your thinking:*

e.g. Hopeful 7/10

_____   _____

_____   _____

_____   _____

_____   _____

_____   _____

_____   _____

Thinking Tools (Part 3) and Relaxation Tools

In Stage 7, you will:

★ learn more about thinking tools in the Emotion Repair Toolbox

★ explore relaxation tools in the Emotion Repair Toolbox.

Activities and Projects for Stage 7
Activities   • Review of Stage 6.   • Self-awareness exercise.   • Challenging negative thoughts.   • Distortions in thinking.   **Projects**   7.1 Writing in your compliments diary.   7.2 Real life practice in recognizing cognitive distortions.   7.3 Adding relaxation time to your weekly planner.   7.4 Self-monitoring.

Review of Stage 6

What is a thinking distortion?

_____

_____

_____

_____

What happens to your mood if you tend to have a lot of thinking distortions?

_____

_____

_____

_____

Why are social tools important?

_____

_____

_____

_____

REVIEW OF YOUR WEEKLY PLAN

Your weekly plan now incorporates four tools in your life, namely physical activities, self-awareness exercises, pleasurable activities and one social activity. You completed a self-monitoring sheet to show when you remembered to do these activities, and also to record how you felt after each of them. Have a look at the self-monitoring sheet now, and answer the following questions:

How did you feel before and after your physical exercise?

_____

_____

_____

_____

What did you schedule as your pleasurable activities?

_____

_____

_____

_____

How is your self-awareness exercise going?

_____

_____

_____

_____

What did you schedule as your social activity?

_____

_____

_____

_____

How did it go?

_____

_____

_____

_____

Self-awareness exercise

Complete a self-awareness exercise now. It will take three to five minutes and will refresh and prepare your mind for the information and activities in Stage 7 (see Appendix I or Appendix III).

Identifying levels of negative emotion

When we are depressed in a particular situation, it is likely that we are experiencing a range of negative emotions or thoughts. For example, we may be miserable, discouraged, depressed, hopeless, jealous, angry, guilty or ashamed.

It is important to understand that emotions and thoughts are not the same things: an emotion is a heightened feeling about someone, yourself or an event; a thought is a belief, idea, intention or expectation. Sometimes it is difficult to distinguish between an emotion and a thought, as they often occur together. But the important point is, we can moderate the intensity of our emotions and thus change our thoughts. This is the technique that is used in the *Exploring Depression* programme.

All of the emotions that we may feel when we are depressed are experienced at different levels of intensity, and thus described slightly differently. In the following table, three different emotions (sadness, anger and anxiety) are broken down in their different levels of intensity, all of which can be identified and named.

Sad	Angry	Anxious
Unhappy	Irritated	Uneasy
Low	Annoyed	Concerned
Downcast	Incensed	Apprehensive
Gloomy	Enraged	Nervous
Disheartened	Fuming	Worried
Miserable	Outraged	Fearful
Bleak	Furious	Frightened
Suicidal	Mad	Panicky

In the following questions, you will be asked to rate the level of intensity of the emotions that you identify.

Challenging negative thoughts

STEP 1

Below, briefly describe a recent situation or event that led to you feeling sad. Were there other negative emotions?

_____

_____

_____

_____

STEP 2

Rate (from the most intense to the least) up to five of the negative emotions you felt at the time. How would you rate each emotion on a scale from 0 to 10 (where 10 is the most intense)?

1. _____ _____

2. _____ _____

3. _____ _____

4. _____ _____

5. _____ _____

STEP 3

Write down the thoughts that came along with each negative emotion you have just described:

	Negative emotion	Thoughts
1.	_____	_____
	_____	_____
2.	_____	_____
	_____	_____
3.	_____	_____
	_____	_____
4.	_____	_____
	_____	_____
5.	_____	_____
	_____	_____

Distortions in thinking

You can refer back to pages 150–152 in Stage 6 to remind yourself about these distortions:

- Black-and-white thinking

- Overgeneralization

- Magical thinking

- Mental filter

- Disqualifying the positive

- Jumping to conclusions

- Magnification and minimization (catastrophizing)

- Emotional reasoning

- 'Should' statements
- Labelling and mislabelling
- Personalization.

STEP 4

Identify the probable distortion in each thought, from the list below:

	Thought	Distortion
1.	_____	_____
2.	_____	_____
3.	_____	_____
4.	_____	_____
5.	_____	_____

STEP 5

Write down a more rational or realistic response to each thought:

	Thought	Rational response
1.	_____	_____
	_____	_____
2.	_____	_____
	_____	_____
3.	_____	_____
	_____	_____
4.	_____	_____
	_____	_____
5.	_____	_____
	_____	_____

STEP 6

Think about the event again, then read your rational responses. What are your negative feelings now when you think of the event? How would you rate each of these emotions, on a scale from 0 to 10 (where 10 is the most intense)?

1. _____ _____

2. _____ _____

3. _____ _____

4. _____ _____

5. _____ _____

Is there a significant reduction in the 'score' for each emotion? (Compare your answers to those in Step 2.)

Have some negative emotions dissolved?

The above six-step activity can be used whenever you encounter an upsetting event that could contribute to your feeling depressed. The more often that you practise these steps, the more realistic and rational you will become, which will in turn decrease the depth of your depression.

Changing the way you think about a situation really can change your feelings.

Identifying relaxation tools

Another tool in the Emotion Repair Toolbox is a relaxation tool. Relaxation tools help you feel calm, prevent you 'catastrophizing' or feeling angry, enable you to carefully consider the situation, and give you time to repair any of the distortions in thinking that were described in Stage 6.

These tools lower your heart rate, induce feelings of well-being and tranquillity and help you to think more clearly, rationally and intelligently.

Relaxation tools can be represented by a paint brush.

Relaxation tools can include: artistic activities such as drawing or listening to music; finding a quiet sanctuary; meditation or yoga; completing routine chores; being in nature or with animals; or reflecting on past, happy experiences.

If you want to develop and enhance the power of relaxation tools, you could learn progressive muscle relaxation[8] or deep relaxation using imagery, or have a regular massage.

The relaxation tools can be divided into those that can be used at home and those you might use at school or work.

List which relaxation tools you use at:

Home   School or work

_____   _____

_____   _____

_____   _____

_____   _____

_____   _____

What relaxation tools have you used successfully in the past but rarely do now?

Home   School or work

_____   _____

_____   _____

_____   _____

_____   _____

_____   _____

---

8   The text for a progressive muscle relaxation is in Appendix V. You can audio record your own voice, or use Michelle or Tony's voices on the downloads available at www.tonyattwood.com.au and www.mindsandhearts.net

What relaxation tools would you like to try for the first time?

       Home   *School or work*

_____   _____

_____   _____

_____   _____

_____   _____

_____   _____

Projects

7.1 Writing in your compliments diary

Continue to record compliments that you have given and received.

7.2 Real life practice in recognizing cognitive distortions

Apply your new knowledge about thinking distortions to a situation that happens between now and when you start the next stage (Stage 8) of the programme.

You can remind yourself of the potential distortions before, during and after the event.

Describe a situation that has led to your feeling sad, angry or anxious:

_____

_____

_____

_____

List any negative emotions that you experienced. Rate the intensity of each emotion on a scale from 0 to 10 (where 10 is the most intense):

_____	_____
_____	_____
_____	_____
_____	_____
_____	_____

Identify the thoughts that came along with the emotions:

Emotion	Thought
_____	_____
_____	_____
_____	_____
_____	_____
_____	_____

Identify the distortions in the thoughts:

Thought	Distortion
_____	_____
_____	_____
_____	_____
_____	_____
_____	_____

Write down a rational response to each thought:

Thought	Rational response
_____	_____
_____	_____
_____	_____
_____	_____
_____	_____

Think about the event again, then read your rational responses.

How do you feel now? Indicate the intensity of each emotion on a scale from 0 to 10:

———————————————————————— ——————————

———————————————————————— ——————————

———————————————————————— ——————————

———————————————————————— ——————————

———————————————————————— ——————————

7.3 Adding relaxation time to your weekly planner

In Stage 7, you will continue to schedule all the activities you included in Stage 6 (i.e. 3–4 physical activities; a daily self-awareness exercise; a daily pleasurable activity; and one social activity), but this time you will also include 2–3 relaxation activities. To remind yourself what activity might be appropriate, refer back to the suggestions you made on pages 174–175. If you would like to do a progressive muscle relaxation, see Appendix IV. Remember, too, that art can also be an excellent relaxation activity, as we discussed in Stage 4.

WEEKLY PLANNER STAGE 7		
Morning	**Afternoon**	**Evening**
Monday		
Tuesday		
Wednesday		
Thursday		
Friday		
Saturday		
Sunday		

Schedule: Physical activities (3–4) Social activity (1)

Self-awareness exercise (daily) Relaxation activities (2–3)

Pleasurable activities (daily)

7.4 Self-monitoring

Use the two, new self-monitoring sheets to record, as before, when you have completed your activities, and also how you felt before and after each one. Also record when you used a thinking tool, and how you felt both before and after the application of this tool. In each case, use the happiness rating scale (0–100).

Your toolbox now comprises many tools, which you are putting into regular practice. You are learning how to reduce the depth of your depression.

SELF-MONITORING (1) STAGE 7

	Self-awareness exercise 1	Physical activity 2	Pleasurable activity 3	Rating (0–100)						
				Before			After			
				1	2	3	1	2	3	
Monday										
Tuesday										
Wednesday										
Thursday										
Friday										
Saturday										
Sunday										

SELF-MONITORING (2) STAGE 7

	Social activity 4	Relaxation activity 5	Thinking tools 6	Rating (0–100) Before			After		
				4	5	6	4	5	6
Monday									
Tuesday									
Wednesday									
Thursday									
Friday									
Saturday									
Sunday									

Relaxation and Helpful and Unhelpful Tools

In Stage 8, you will:

★ learn to use a relaxation tool for self-awareness

★ discover other helpful tools

★ identify unhelpful tools.

Activities and Projects for Stage 8

Activities

- Review of Stage 7.

- Self-awareness exercise.

- Relaxation for self-awareness.

Projects

8.1 Writing in your compliments diary.

8.2 Adding another relaxation or art activity to your weekly planner.

8.3 Self-monitoring.

8.4 Applying your key strengths to achieve greater success in a chosen area of your life.

8.5 Recording your level of sadness during the last week.

Review of Stage 7

Which thinking distortion do you tend to use more than others?

_____

_____

_____

_____

What is the benefit of relaxation?

_____

_____

_____

_____

Why would this help to alleviate depression?

_____

_____

_____

_____

REVIEW OF YOUR WEEKLY PLAN

You continued to follow a weekly plan that incorporated five tools into your life, namely, physical activities, self-awareness exercises, pleasurable activities, a social activity and a relaxation activity. You also completed self-monitoring sheets to record when you had remembered to do these activities, and also to record how you felt after each of them. Have a look at the two self-monitoring sheets now, and answer the following questions:

How did you feel before and after your physical exercise?

_____

_____

_____

_____

What did you schedule as your pleasurable activity?

_____

_____

_____

_____

How is your self-awareness exercise going?

_____

_____

_____

_____

EXPLORING DEPRESSION, AND BEATING THE BLUES

What did you schedule as your social activity?

_____

_____

_____

_____

Did you enjoy parts of your social activity? What would have made your social activity more enjoyable? What did you learn about yourself?

_____

_____

_____

_____

What did you schedule for your relaxation activity?

_____

_____

_____

_____

Were you able to experience relaxation? If not, in your opinion what could have helped you to achieve greater relaxation?

_____

_____

_____

_____

You applied your new knowledge about thinking distortions to enable you to understand your feelings about an event or thought over the previous week. What happened?

_____

_____

_____

_____

Were there any barriers to using this strategy? What were these? How could you overcome them?

_____

_____

_____

_____

Self-awareness exercise

Complete a self-awareness exercise now (see Appendix I or Appendix III). It will take three to five minutes and will help you to move into Stage 8 of the programme with a clear, focused mind.

Relaxation for self-awareness

For this exercise you will need to use the download entitled *Relaxation for Self-awareness* that comes with this programme.[9] If for any reason this is not available to you, use the text, which you can find in Appendix VII, for the activity. You can audio record the text, and then listen back to it to complete the activity.

Settle yourself comfortably in your chair. Listen to the audio recording of *Relaxation for Self-awareness*, which is an exercise for your mind to help you both relax and discover more aspects of yourself.

Once you have completed the activity, take a moment to reflect on your experience. Describe your own experience of success or achievement:

_____

_____

_____

_____

List your key strengths that enabled you to succeed:

_____

_____

_____

_____

How did your key strengths contribute to your success?

_____

_____

_____

_____

---

9 See 'Downloads for Exploring Depression' at www.tonyattwood.com.au and www.mindsandhearts.net

Other helpful tools in the Emotion Repair Toolbox

Medication

As discussed in Chapter 4 of this programme, medication can be a successful treatment for depression. Medication is most helpful when used in conjunction with an empirically validated psychotherapy, such as the programme that you are following in this book. If you have taken medication before for depression or anxiety, consider the following questions:

What have been the good aspects of medication?

_____

_____

_____

_____

What have been your concerns?

_____

_____

_____

_____

If you wish to find out more about medication for depression or anxiety, we recommend talking to your general practitioner or psychiatrist.

Religious, spiritual or personal beliefs

Exploring aspects of religious, spiritual or personal beliefs can alleviate depression and encourage a feeling of well-being, optimism and happiness. If you belong to a particular religion, it may be worthwhile discussing your feelings and sense of depression with a senior member of that religion or spiritual group.

Nutrition

Advice from mature adults who have Asperger's syndrome is that good nutrition can have a significant, beneficial effect on mood. Information about diet and nutrition is not within the scope of this programme. However, it may be worthwhile your seeing a dietitian for advice on how changing aspects of your diet could improve both your physical and mental health.

Sleep

Typically, people with Asperger's syndrome have difficulty falling asleep and often have concerns with regard to the inadequate duration, depth and quality of their sleep. Consequently, there is a risk of chronic sleep deprivation. This inevitably has serious consequences for both physical and mental health. An assessment at a sleep clinic may provide valuable information and advice on how to achieve a quality of sleep that has a positive effect on energy levels, mood and general well-being.

Having a caring role

Being a volunteer for those who need help, or caring for animals or pets can be effective strategies to help overcome depression. Being needed and appreciated is a powerful antidote to feeling lonely and depressed, and can be a major reason why suicidal thoughts, if they occur at all, remain just that – thoughts.

Are there any other helpful tools you have discovered that we have not explored? List these below:

_____

_____

_____

_____

Unhelpful tools

Some tools for dealing with depression are not recommended. These include taking illegal drugs or misusing prescription drugs; using alcohol; injuring yourself; or hurting someone else, either verbally or physically.

Alcohol or drugs

Sometimes people with Asperger's syndrome start to use alcohol or other mind-altering substances, such as marijuana, opiates or amphetamines, to try to gain relief from feeling anxious or depressed. Initially, the associated feelings of relaxation, and the creation of a barrier or emotional detachment from aspects of life that are depressing or hurtful, can lead to the person continuing to increase the quantity of alcohol and drugs, such that they come to rely exclusively on such substances to cope with feeling depressed.

In our modern society, alcohol and drugs are more available than ever before. Research and our clinical experience would suggest that between ten and 30 per cent of patients at drug and alcohol treatment and rehabilitation services have the characteristics of Asperger's syndrome. Why would those who have Asperger's syndrome choose the path of addiction in their later adolescence or young adult years?

There are many reasons. The pathway usually starts with access to alcohol, a socially acceptable, but very potent drug. For the person who has Asperger's syndrome, alcohol can initially appear to remove the barriers of social inhibition, and facilitate social cohesion and inclusion. Alcohol can also reduce social anxiety and the fear of making a *faux pas*. It can facilitate the creation of a new, more popular character. It provides a sense of emotional detachment and imperviousness to derogatory remarks, and creates an emotional shield or protective 'bubble'; and often, it offers the possibility of inclusion and acceptance in a marginalized peer group of fellow alcohol and drug users.

The next stage can be to experiment with a range of illegal drugs and prescription medication, potentially leading to an addiction. The consequences of intoxication can include being less able to access the frontal lobes, or the thinking and planning areas of the brain, and increased difficulties processing social information, thus actually amplifying the central characteristics of Asperger's syndrome. With reduced frontal lobe abilities, the person may also make impulsive or unwise decisions, leading to risky behaviour. There is also the risk of being in conflict with the law and entering the criminal justice system. In addition, and importantly, most recreational drugs, such as alcohol and marijuana, directly contribute to the biochemistry and thought processes associated with depression.

Self-harm

The use of self-harm, for example cutting, burning or otherwise injuring oneself, can sometimes be the consequence of a need to feel something because of a pervasive sense of emotional numbness, a need to feel physical pain to block out emotional pain or to create a sense of relaxation. Endorphins are released at the time of cutting, which can lead to the person wishing to continue to cut or hurt themselves. It is very important if this is happening for you that you seek professional help.

Self-harming can be very dangerous, and it is important that you are monitored and assisted to learn new ways to manage your difficult and intense emotions. Contact your general practitioner, psychiatrist or psychologist to seek understanding and help.

Many of the tools and strategies discussed in this programme will be ones that you can learn to use in order to replace the need to self-harm.

Hurting someone else

Particularly when we are angry (and anger can be an expression of depression, as discussed in Chapter 3), it can be tension-relieving and satisfying to hurt someone else, either physically or verbally. Clearly, in calmer moments we can reflect that hurting someone else is never a good idea, nor is it an appropriate way to express despair, discharging it like an emotional 'bolt of lightning'.

First of all, considerable damage can occur to the relationship with the person you have harmed, which can lead to the end of that relationship.

Second, to live happily in the world we need to live with ourselves and what we do, and the remorse, guilt, shame and regret we feel after hurting someone else is very harmful to us, and could deepen and prolong the depression.

Third, hurting someone else can lead to being in conflict with the law, such as domestic violence orders, hefty fines, or even imprisonment. Continuing to rely on the tool of hurting someone else is extremely harmful, both to you and to the person involved. For any perceived short-term benefit, there is a far greater and painful long-term cost to be considered.

Are there other 'tools' that you have used that were not wise decisions or actions?

_____

_____

_____

_____

Have you used any tools that were potentially harmful to a relationship or led to conflict with the law?

_____

_____

_____

_____

What tools have you used that made the depression worse?

_____

_____

_____

_____

Projects

8.1 Writing in your compliments diary

Continue to record compliments that you have given and received.

8.2 Adding another relaxation or art activity to your weekly planner

Now at Stage 8, you will schedule an extra relaxation or art activity (see Stage 7) into your weekly plan. Continue to schedule all other activities as you did previously.

WEEKLY PLANNER STAGE 8		
Morning	Afternoon	Evening
Monday		
Tuesday		
Wednesday		
Thursday		
Friday		
Saturday		
Sunday		

Schedule: Physical activities (3–4) Social activity (1)
Self-awareness exercise (daily) Relaxation activities (2–3)
Pleasurable activities (daily)

8.3 Self-monitoring

Use the two self-monitoring sheets to record, as you did before, when you have completed your activities and exercises, and also how you felt before and after each one. Record when you used a thinking tool, and how you felt both before and after the application of this tool. In each case, use the happiness rating scale (0–100).

SELF-MONITORING (1) STAGE 8

	Self-awareness exercise 1	Physical activity 2	Pleasurable activity 3	Rating (0–100)						
				Before			After			
				1	2	3	1	2	3	
Monday										
Tuesday										
Wednesday										
Thursday										
Friday										
Saturday										
Sunday										

SELF-MONITORING (2) STAGE 8

	Social activity 4	Relaxation activity 5	Thinking tools 6	Rating (0–100)					
				Before			After		
				4	5	6	4	5	6
Monday									
Tuesday									
Wednesday									
Thursday									
Friday									
Saturday									
Sunday									

8.4 Applying your key strengths to achieve greater success in a chosen area of your life

Within which area of your life would you like to gain more success?

_____

_____

_____

_____

What are your key strengths? (Refer to notes from Stages 1 and 8 as needed.)

_____

_____

_____

_____

How can you apply your strengths in your chosen area?

_____

_____

_____

_____

Important last step:
Take some time to relax. Imagine a positive and successful future using these strengths.

8.5 Recording your level of sadness during the last week

Have you had any of the thoughts listed below in the last week? If you have, can you indicate with an x whether you have had them not at all, sometimes (once or twice) or often (three times or more).

	Not at all	Sometimes	Often
I am a failure	☐	☐	☐
My life will never get better	☐	☐	☐
Nobody likes me	☐	☐	☐
People are disappointed in me	☐	☐	☐
I disappoint myself	☐	☐	☐
I can't change	☐	☐	☐
What would it be like if I were dead?	☐	☐	☐
I want to be alone and just cry	☐	☐	☐

Your answers will be explored in Stage 9.

A Safety Plan

In Stage 9, you will learn:

★ to measure the depth of your sadness, enabling you to decide which repair tool to use at each level

★ to manage the deepest level of sadness, a 'depression attack'.

Activities and Projects for Stage 9

Activities

• Review of Stage 8.

• Self-awareness exercise.

• Deciding which tools to use to repair the different levels of sadness.

• Understanding and managing desperate despair.

Projects

9.1 Sharing your safety plan.

9.2 Identifying the ways in which you would like to achieve more success.

9.3 Writing in your compliments diary.

9.4 Filling in your weekly planner.

9.5 Self-monitoring.

Review of Stage 8

Which successful experience did you reflect on during the relaxation exercise?

_____

_____

_____

_____

Which of your own strengths allowed you to make that experience a success?

_____

_____

_____

_____

Which tools are not wise or effective in the long term for emotion repair when you feel sad or depressed?

_____

_____

_____

_____

REVIEW OF YOUR WEEKLY PLAN

In Stage 8, you followed a plan that incorporated five tools into your life, including an extra relaxation or art activity. You completed two self-monitoring sheets, recording when you did these activities, and also how you felt having completed each of them. You also recorded when you used your thinking tools. Have a look at the two self-monitoring sheets now, and answer the following questions:

How did you feel before and after your physical exercise?

_____

_____

_____

_____

How is your self-awareness exercise going?

_____

_____

_____

_____

How are your pleasurable activities going?

_____

_____

_____

_____

What did you schedule as your social activity?

_____

_____

_____

_____

How did it go?

_____

_____

_____

_____

What did you schedule for your relaxation activities?

_____

_____

_____

_____

How did they go?

_____

_____

_____

_____

Were you able to relax and imagine a positive and successful future based on your qualities and strengths?

_____

_____

What is that future?

_____

_____

_____

_____

Reflect for a moment on how sad you felt in the last week. How sad did you feel overall on a scale from 0–10, with 10 being the most sad?

Level of sadness _____

Self-awareness exercise

Complete your self-awareness exercise now (see Appendix I or Appendix III). It will take three to five minutes and will refresh and prepare your mind for the activities of Stage 9.

Deciding which tools to use to repair the different levels of sadness

In Stage 2 you were introduced to the concept of a thermometer to measure the 'temperature', or intensity, of sad feelings. Below is the diagram of that thermometer, listing, as before, the words that describe the different levels of intensity of sadness and despair. You may want to change the words to those that you prefer to use yourself.

In Stage 2, you explored the reasons for the various levels of sadness. This time, write on the right hand side the specific tools from your Emotion Repair Toolbox that could fix or repair the various levels of sadness:

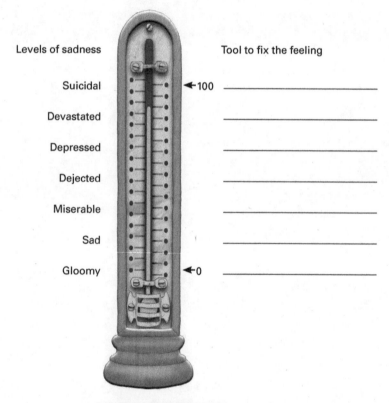

Levels of sadness | Tool to fix the feeling

Suicidal ← 100 _____

Devastated _____

Depressed _____

Dejected _____

Miserable _____

Sad _____

Gloomy ← 0 _____

SADNESS THERMOMETER

Understanding and managing desperate despair

SELF-HARM AND SUICIDAL THOUGHTS

Over the last year, have you ever been so desperately sad that you have deliberately harmed yourself?

Yes ☐   No ☐

Over the last year, have you ever been so desperately sad that you have thought of ending your life?

Yes ☐   No ☐

There is a difference between briefly thinking about suicide as a concept or option, and actually having detailed thoughts how to end your life. If you have seriously thought of ending your life, why did you think that death would be a solution?

_____

_____

_____

_____

What made you decide not to end your life?

_____

_____

_____

_____

REACHING OUT FOR HELP

If you have those thoughts again, it is important to have a constructive strategy to alleviate feeling so desperately and dangerously sad that you consider suicide. An important constructive strategy is to disclose the depth of your feelings to someone who can help you move through and out of the depths of despair.

You may be reluctant to tell this person, as you do not want to upset them or make them worry about you, but *someone needs to know* so that together you can end the depth of despair.

To whom could you disclose your experiences of self-harm or suicidal feelings?

_____

_____

_____

_____

How would you want them to help you?

1. _____
2. _____
3. _____
4. _____
5. _____

What strategies have you used in the past to recover from feeling so desperately sad?

1. _____
2. _____
3. _____
4. _____
5. _____

What new strategies have you learnt in the stages of this programme that you could use in the future?

1. _____

2. _____

3. _____

4. _____

5. _____

Developing a safety plan for suicidal thoughts and actions

A 'depression attack'

The stresses of your life can gradually intensify without you being consciously aware of them, or of the resultant increasing pressure. Then, a relatively minor negative event can occur and the pressure, as in a balloon, goes 'pop'; you may have sudden, unexpected and extremely intense feelings of utter despair. The negative feelings are overwhelming, an emotional 'implosion' occurs and there appear to be no solutions that you can think of for your overwhelming problems. There is just a desperate need to stop the feelings, and you may consider ending your life as a compelling solution.

We describe a catastrophic and extremely intense experience of depression as a 'depression attack'.

Depression attacks usually arrive unexpectedly and are extremely intense, but they also tend to end quickly. This can be very confusing to other people, but it is important to remember that the 'attack' can actually be brief and gone almost as quickly as it appeared. You may have experienced depression attacks before. We have known of children who have Asperger's syndrome experiencing their first depression attacks in their primary school years. Please remember that these are intense, but relatively brief, experiences, and you have lived through them all so far, to tell the tale.

While the feelings are very real and unbearable, there are strategies to make the despair less intense and to prevent actions during the attack that are dangerous and life threatening.

Strategies for dealing with a depression attack
Strategies for you
You must:

- Immediately seek practical or emotional help, from a trusted family member, friend teacher or colleague. This is an emotional emergency.

- Try to remove yourself from the situation that triggered the depression attack.

- Try not to injure yourself.

- Try using thoughts about, or engage in, your special interest as an 'off switch', distraction and barrier to feeling intense despair.

Strategies for your support person
The following are strategies that someone can use to help you while you are experiencing a depression attack. Your support person should:

- *Stay calm and reassuring*: The agitation or confusion of another person will intensify your depth of despair, adding 'fuel to the fire'. You may make hurtful comments, but the person helping you move through and out of the depression attack must not express their own distress in response to your comments and actions.

- *Not ask what is causing the distress*: In such an intense emotional state, insight and coherent explanations are elusive and trying to explain and re-enter the experience may make the situation worse. It is more important to move on through and out of the depression attack.

- *Stay with you*: Left alone, there is the risk for you of an impulsive action that could be dangerous. For safety reasons, someone needs to see you and be able to protect you from yourself or any destructive action. They do not have to be physically close, but within the same room or just several metres away.

- *Not try to 'fix the problem'*: Such intense emotions prevent the acceptance of suggestions which, at this stage of despair, will almost certainly be rejected, and perceived as provocative and lacking understanding and appreciation of the problem.

- *Not move in too close without prior approval*: Encroaching uninvited into your personal body space, perhaps to express affection or compassion, may cause a physical reaction of rejection, such that they could be pushed away and be physically hurt. Affection may be used in such circumstances, but only with your prior approval, and at a level of expression that is soothing rather than confusing or overwhelming.

- *Validate the feelings and just listen*: You may need to express your despair in words and expletives. This helps you to release the intense emotion. Your listener needs to acknowledge your feelings in a non-judgemental way, even if he or she does not agree with them. For example, he or she may say to you, 'I know and appreciate how you feel completely hopeless and in such despair right now.'

- *Remind you that the intense despair will go*: One of the characteristics of a 'depression attack' is that it is usually of short duration. You can be reassured that the feeling will eventually go.

- *Engage in minimal conversation*: This is not the time for a conversation, on any topic, as a distraction. The ending of the depression attack will come from within you. You need to withdraw from conversation and any social interaction in order to focus all mental energy on recovery.

- *Find a quiet sanctuary you can share to relax*: There is a clear need to retreat to a safe sanctuary, without social, conversational or sensory demands. Neither should there be criticism, disappointment, anger or fear as to what you may be thinking or might do.

- *Avoid intense eye contact*: Having someone stare into your eyes whilst you are enduring a depression attack, especially with an intense facial expression, will probably create greater despair or confusion. It may be wise for your support person to look at your shoulder, or about a metre to the side of you.

- *Encourage participation in a special interest if you feel able*: This can be the 'off switch' to provide an intellectual distraction, restore constructive rather than destructive energy, and enable a feeling of familiarity and well-being.

- *Allow time to process the intense emotions*: The restoration of an emotional equilibrium may be a solitary process, with time to process thoughts, events and emotions before being able to move on to a new, positive frame of mind.

Which of these strategies would help you when you are feeling intense despair?

_____

_____

_____

_____

_____

_____

Create a plan to manage a future depression attack:

_____

_____

_____

_____

_____

_____

_____

_____

You could write or type the plan to manage your depression attack on a blank business card, and have several copies of the card with you. You may give a card to someone who is supporting you when a depression attack occurs. During the intense despair, you may not be able to fluently and coherently articulate the strategies you need during this depression crisis, and the card will provide clear guidelines on what that person can do to help. The card may also have the phone number of someone to contact for further advice on how to manage the situation or to talk to you.

Try visualizing the experience of a depression attack as being on a gigantic roller-coaster ride. It may feel dangerous, but it is only truly dangerous if you jump out of the cart. Eventually the momentum will cease, and you will return to the starting point. Only then can you safely leave the cart.

Projects

9.1 Sharing your safety plan

Share your safety plan with your family, friends or colleagues – those who need to know what to do to help you.

Make sure your safety plan is easily available and remembered. Almost as they would with a fire drill, your family or friends may need to be reminded and regularly practise what to do.

9.2 Identifying the ways in which you would like to achieve more success

Identify an area of your life where you would like to be more successful. It could be a desire to make a good friend, or to have a better quality of friendship or relationships than you currently have, or a better relationship with your parents or siblings.

It may be you would like to be more successful at school, college or work.

Write down the areas in your life where you would like to be more successful in the future:

_____

_____

_____

_____

Think about how you can apply your key strengths in personality and ability (identified in Stages 1 and 2) to be more successful in the area of life that you have chosen.

Write down any ideas that you have to use your qualities or key strengths:

_____

_____

_____

_____

_____

_____

_____

9.3 Writing in your compliments diary

Continue to record compliments that you have given and received.

9.4 Filling in your weekly planner

Your busy, productive schedule continues in Stage 9, with the same activities and exercises that you did in Stage 8: daily self-awareness exercises and pleasurable activities, three or four physical activities, two or three relaxation activities or exercises, and one social activity.

WEEKLY PLANNER STAGE 9		
Morning	Afternoon	Evening
Monday		
Tuesday		
Wednesday		
Thursday		
Friday		
Saturday		
Sunday		

Schedule: Physical activities (3–4) Social activity (1)

Self-awareness exercise (daily) Relaxation activities (2–3)

Pleasurable activities (daily)

9.5 Self-monitoring

Use the two self-monitoring sheets to record, as before, when you have completed your activities and exercises, and again rate how you felt before and after each one. Record when you used a thinking tool, and how you felt both before and after the application of this tool. In each case, use the happiness rating scale (0–100).

SELF-MONITORING (1) STAGE 9

	Self-awareness exercise 1	Physical activity 2	Pleasurable activity 3	Rating (0–100)					
				Before			After		
				1	2	3	1	2	3
Monday									
Tuesday									
Wednesday									
Thursday									
Friday									
Saturday									
Sunday									

SELF-MONITORING (2) STAGE 9

	Social activity 4	Relaxation activity 5	Thinking tools 6	Rating (0–100)					
				Before			After		
				4	5	6	4	5	6
Monday									
Tuesday									
Wednesday									
Thursday									
Friday									
Saturday									
Sunday									

The Future

In Stage 10, you will:

★ imagine the sort of life you want for the future

★ plan how to get the life you want, using your increasing self-awareness, strengths in personality and abilities and the tools you have explored in this programme

★ review the programme.

Activities and Projects for Stage 10

Activities

- Review of Stage 9.
- Self-awareness exercise.
- Time machine: Imagining the life you want.
- Planning how to have the life you want.
- Programme review.

Projects

10.1 Filling in your weekly planner.

102. Self-monitoring.

Review of Stage 9

What is your safety plan for when you may experience a depression attack?

_____

_____

_____

_____

Which emotion repair tools could you use?

_____

_____

_____

_____

REVIEW OF YOUR WEEKLY PLAN

As before, you followed your schedule that incorporated five important tools into your life. You also completed two self-monitoring sheets to record when you did these five activities, and how you felt before and after completing them. Take a look at the two self-monitoring sheets now, reflect on your experience and ask yourself these questions:

How did you feel before and after your physical exercise?

_____

_____

_____

_____

How is your self-awareness exercise going?

_____

_____

_____

_____

What did you schedule as your social activity?

_____

_____

_____

_____

How did it go?

_____

_____

_____

_____

What did you schedule for your pleasurable activities?

_____

_____

_____

_____

How did your pleasurable activities go?

_____

_____

_____

_____

What did you schedule for your relaxation activity?

_____

_____

_____

_____

How did your relaxation activity go?

_____

_____

_____

_____

What were your parents' and friends' or colleagues' thoughts on your safety plan?

_____

_____

_____

_____

Which area of your life would you like to be more successful?

_____

_____

_____

_____

Self-awareness exercise

Complete your self-awareness exercise now (see Appendix I or Appendix III). It will take three to five minutes and will result in a clear, focused mind for the new learning involved in Stage 10 of the programme.

Time machine: Imagining the life you want

During this activity, you will use relaxation and imagery to imagine a celebration in your life in about ten years' time. There is an audio recording for Stage 10, entitled *Time Machine Activity*. Download this audio recording now,[10] or audio record the text in Appendix VII to use during this activity. Choose a time to complete this activity when you are feeling relatively positive about your life. It is harder to do it when you are feeling bleak, as it can be very difficult to envisage an improvement in your circumstances, level of happiness and sense of self at these times.

You will be asked to imagine a celebration of an achievement that you have yearned for. There will be people there that you know now, and new people that you have welcomed into your life. You will consider where you are living, the work or study you are doing, the qualifications you have achieved and who is important in your life.

Listen to the audio recording now, and answer the following questions.

Where were you living?

_____

_____

_____

_____

What work or study were you doing?

_____

_____

_____

_____

10 See 'Downloads for Exploring Depression' at www.mindsandhearts.net or www.tonyattwood.com.au

Who was important in your life?

_____

_____

_____

_____

Planning how to have the life you want

Knowing *what you want* from life is a necessary goal. How do you reach a goal if you do not know want you are aiming for?

Knowing *how to get there* is also necessary. You will need a plan, abilities and qualities, and your emotion repair tools ready to use if you need them.

THE PLAN

As with many of the activities suggested throughout this programme, it is strongly recommended that, in this important phase of planning for your future, you seek guidance and assistance from someone that you trust, or from a professional trained for this work, for example, a clinical psychologist or a life coach.

What is your goal? (Note: It is most helpful if your goal is aligned with your personal values, abilities, qualities and skills. Try to make your goal realistic to give yourself the best opportunity to succeed.)

_____

_____

_____

_____

When would you like to have achieved this goal by?

_____

_____

_____

_____

IDENTIFYING ABILITIES

Which abilities do you have that will help you get where you want to go?

_____

_____

_____

_____

Which abilities and skills do you need to have, that you do not have right now?

_____

_____

_____

_____

How can you learn or acquire these abilities and skills?

_____

_____

_____

_____

IDENTIFYING PERSONAL QUALITIES

Which personal qualities do you have that will help you get where you want to go?

_____

_____

_____

_____

Which personality qualities do you not have that you may need to reach your goal?

_____

_____

_____

_____

How can you cultivate the personality qualities that you will need to achieve your goal?

_____

_____

_____

_____

IDENTIFYING THE STEPS TO SUCCESS

Who are your allies (that is, the people who will support you in this goal)?

_____

_____

_____

_____

Write down the steps, as you envision them, which you need to take in order to reach your goal.

1. _____

2. _____

3. _____

4. _____

5. _____

6. _____

7. _____

8. _____

9. _____

10. _____

What barriers might you encounter along the way?

_____

_____

_____

_____

What strategies can you employ to overcome these barriers?

_____

_____

_____

_____

IDENTIFYING THE TOOLS FOR THE JOURNEY

You will have discovered, through your own practice and from this programme, the tools that have been most helpful to you. On a scale from 0 to 10, rate how helpful each has been, with 10 being the most helpful. Add your own comments.

- *Self-awareness tools*

  Rating _____

  Comment:

  _____

  _____

- *Physical tools*

  Rating _____

  Comment:

  _____

  _____

- *Pleasure tools*

  Rating _____

  Comment:

  _____

  _____

- *Thinking tools*

  Rating _____

  Comment:

  _____

  _____

- *Social tools*

  Rating _____

  Comment:

  _____

  _____

- *Relaxation tools*

  Rating _____

  Comment:

  _____

  _____

There may be some tools that you felt might have worked but that you did not get to try very much.

Which tools were these?

_____

_____

_____

_____

What were the barriers to trying them?

_____

_____

_____

_____

Programme review

What did you find most helpful about the programme?

_____

_____

_____

_____

What was least helpful?

_____

_____

_____

_____

How could the programme be improved?

_____

_____

_____

_____

What steps could you take to make this programme work better for you?

_____

_____

_____

_____

Assessing and maintaining your progress

Congratulations on all your hard work! You have now completed the ten component stages of the *Exploring Depression* programme.

Assessment

It is now time to complete two of the assessments that you completed at the very start of the programme, in Chapter 7. Go back to this chapter now, complete Assessments 2 and 3 (the DASS and 'Imaginary Scene'), and then compare your original results with your results now.

Assessment 2: DASS

Previous DASS score _____

Current DASS score _____

Assessment 3: Imaginary Scene

Suggested strategies:

_____

_____

_____

_____

_____

_____

_____

_____

Previous number of suggested strategies: _____

Current number of suggested strategies: _____

It is highly likely, if you have been motivated, and followed the programme with a positive and determined attitude, that, even if you have not completed every single activity or project, you will have noticed a significant improvement in your mood and, as a result of this programme and your hard work, you will have obtained a level of well-being that was not available to you before you started the programme.

If you do not feel there has been a significant improvement in your mood, please ask a family member or friend if they have noticed an improvement. They may have noticed changes that you are perhaps not aware of. If there is general agreement that the signs of depression are as great as they ever were, then it would be appropriate to seek professional help from a clinician who specializes in the treatment of depression.

Maintaining the positive gains

Should you have made the hoped-for positive gains during the programme, then maintaining the gains will be the next challenge! You now have the resources you need, including information about important emotion repair tools that you can use, and your weekly planners and self-monitoring sheets to monitor your progress. We encourage you to continue to monitor your progress for another four weeks at least as the final stage of the programme. After this time, it is fine to discontinue the use of your weekly planners and self-monitoring sheets if you wish to. It is likely that, at this stage of the programme, your good lifestyle habits will continue because they are self-rewarding.

We sincerely hope that this is your outcome. However, if it is not your outcome and you have tried your very best to complete the programme, we strongly recommend that you seek additional assistance. We encourage you to reach out to a general practitioner, or clinical psychologist or psychiatrist, for further assistance.

Relapse prevention

Sometimes a relapse may occur, where you start to experience a build-up of the old feelings of sadness and depression. If this happens to you, the best strategy is to acknowledge it early, rather than denying that it is happening.

Relapse is not a sign of weakness or failure, and is common in both anxiety and depression. It is important to recognize any signs of relapse, and use these as a reminder to reinvigorate your knowledge and employ your tools and strategies again. It may be time to go through this self-help guide again.

Keeping a mood diary

Feelings of sadness tend to fluctuate from day to day as a reaction to specific events, but can also fluctuate according to internal cycles, or 'tides', of depression. This is an underlying sadness that is not simply a reaction to events in your life, but slowly-gathering feelings of low mood over days, weeks or months.

We have developed the concept of a mood diary to record your daily level of overall mood to forewarn of any depression cycles. The process is very simple but can provide invaluable data to prevent a relapse into depression (see Appendix VIII).

At the end of each day, reflect on how you felt on a dimension of happy to sad and the other dimensions of relaxed to anxious, affection to anger and smart to stupid. With regard to the depression dimension, you can use a numerical rating from zero to twenty, with ten being your usual or default level of contentment. Zero to nine would be the sad to depressed range, with zero being feelings of severe depression and nine being just a little down or morose. Eleven to twenty would be the happy range, with eleven being a little more content than usual and twenty being a sense of euphoria.

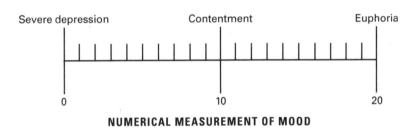

NUMERICAL MEASUREMENT OF MOOD

Each day, decide the single numerical rating that measures your overall level or position on the dimension of sadness to happiness. Record that level in a diary and then create a chart or graph with the horizontal axis being time (days) and the vertical axis being the rating (0 to 20). Gradually, a pattern or trend may become apparent that can indicate that a relapse is impending and that you will need to refresh your strategies and protect you from becoming depressed again.

It is important to record your moods over time, even if, at the time of recording, you are feeling very down and you have your lowest level of energy. It takes only a moment to use the above scale, and you may feel better for engaging in this quick and simple activity which can act as a cue to engage in emotional repair.

Mood

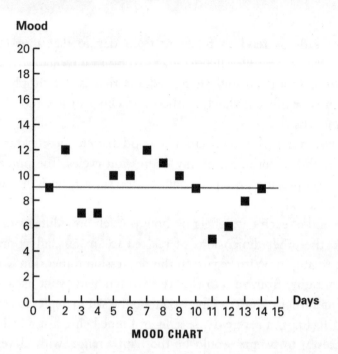

MOOD CHART

There will be occasional exceptions to the trend, due to particular events, such as the death of someone you know, or a pet; or you might experience an especially happy or successful event, such as achieving a particularly high mark in an exam, or promotion to a position that you have always wanted to achieve; but you may start to recognize that your mood fluctuates for a variety of other reasons. For some people, the time of the year, such as the depth of winter, can increase the level of sadness. It is also recognized that both the lunar and menstrual cycles can have significant effects on mood. And some people find that they have an ability to cope with life for a defined duration, but regularly, after a specified time, say seven to nine weeks, there is a temporary sadness crash.

At the first sign of the old feelings of depression returning, we recommend that you complete an assessment of your depression: see Chapter 7 of this programme. Next, revisit Tools for the Journey (pages 228–229) to remind yourself of your own most helpful and powerful strategies and tools to beat the blues.

If it is caught in the early stages, the relapse can be less severe and easier to remedy.

Projects
10.1 Filling in your weekly planner

Take out your new planning sheet for the week. Think about the times in the coming weeks that you can schedule in your usual activities that you have been including for the past few weeks (see the list at the bottom of the planner).

WEEKLY PLANNER STAGE 10		
	Morning	Afternoon	Evening
Monday			
Tuesday			
Wednesday			
Thursday			
Friday			
Saturday			
Sunday			

Schedule: Physical activities (3–4) Social activity (1)
Self-awareness exercise (daily) Relaxation or art activities (2–3)
Pleasurable activities (daily)

10.2 Self-monitoring

Use the two self-monitoring sheets to record, as usual, when you completed all your activities, and how you felt before and after each one (0–100).

SELF-MONITORING (1) STAGE 10

	Self-awareness exercise 1	Physical activity 2	Pleasurable activity 3	Rating (0–100)						
				Before			After			
				1	2	3	1	2	3	
Monday										
Tuesday										
Wednesday										
Thursday										
Friday										
Saturday										
Sunday										

SELF-MONITORING (2) STAGE 10

	Social activity 4	Relaxation activity 5	Thinking tools 6	Rating (0–100)					
				Before			After		
				4	5	6	4	5	6
Monday									
Tuesday									
Wednesday									
Thursday									
Friday									
Saturday									
Sunday									

Managing your time in the future

Remember, you may choose to continue to use planners and self-monitoring sheets for a while, or you may find that you have now become familiar enough with your activities to be able to manage your time without visual reminders. You can always come back to them in the future, should you need to.

Recommended Reading

Attwood, T., Evans, C.R., and Lesko, A. (2014) *Been There. Done That. Try This! An Aspie's Guide to Life on Earth.* London: Jessica Kingsley Publishers.

Dubin, N. (2014) *The Autism Spectrum and Depression.* London: Jessica Kingsley Publishers.

Schab, L.M. (2008) *Beyond the Blues: A Workbook to Help Teens Overcome Depression.* Oakland, CA: Instant Help Books.

Skov, V. (2015) *Integrative Art Therapy and Depression: A Transformative Approach.* London: Jessica Kingsley Publishers.

Wilkinson, L.A. (2015) *Overcoming Anxiety and Depression on the Autism Spectrum: A Self-Help Guide Using CBT.* London: Jessica Kingsley Publishers.

Recommended Websites

American Psychological Association: Understanding depression and effective treatment

www.apa.org/helpcenter/understanding-depression.aspx

Information on the causes of depression and psychological treatment options for recovery.

Anxiety and Depression Association of America

www.adaa.org/finding-help/getting-support/support-groups/online-phone

Directory of recommended support groups.

Beyond Blue

www.beyondblue.org.au

Support and advice on depression and anxiety.

Black Dog Institute

www.blackdoginstitute.org.au

A not-for-profit organisation working on the diagnosis, treatment and prevention of mood disorders.

Depression Comix

www.depressioncomix.com

Single-panel comics on depression.

headspace

http://headspace.org.au

For people aged 12–25 and their families.

MensLine Australia

www.mensline.org.au

For men facing mental health or relationship issues.

Mind

www.mind.org.uk

Mental health charity providing help to make choices about treatment and sources of support.

mindhealthconnect

www.mindhealthconnect.org.au

A source of trusted mental health and wellbeing information, online programmes, helplines and news.

The National Autistic Society: Mental health and autism

www.autism.org.uk/about/health/mental-health.aspx

An article on anxiety disorder, OCD and depression in people with autism.

NHS Choices: Depression support groups

www.nhs.uk/conditions/stress-anxiety-depression/pages/depression-help-groups.aspx

Recommends self-help support groups and other types of depression support.

Q Life

https://qlife.org.au

For support for people who are LGBTI.

SANE: Depression

www.sane.org.uk/resources/mental_health_conditions/depression

Information on and support services for people suffering from depression.

SupportLine

www.supportline.org.uk/problems/depression.php

Provides a confidential telephone helpline offering emotional support, as well as other sources of support.

Bringing the Body into Awareness

Take some time to settle yourself into your chair.

Sit with both feet on the floor, eyes gently closed or looking into the middle distance.

Rest your hands on your lap, or your forearms on the arms of the chair – whichever is more comfortable.

Start to become aware of your breath. Notice the in breath...and the out breath...the in breath...and the out breath...

Become aware of being in your body now.

Notice the sensation of your feet on the floor, the slight sense of pressure as your feet rest on the ground. Notice the chair under your legs, on the backs of your thighs, the touch of the chair on your back, and perhaps on the backs of your upper arms and forearms. Become aware of the sensation of your clothes on your skin: the light touch of fabric on your torso, the lower half of your body... Now start to notice the light touch of air on your skin...your face...the backs of your hands.

Gently bring your attention back to the breath. Without seeking to change the breath, observe the breath as it enters the body, and exits the body. In and out...in... out...

And now I want you to imagine that you are sitting right inside your mind...in the middle, where it is safe, dark and warm. Shortly I am going to be asking you to move your attention through each part of your body. When we do this, I would like you to imagine that your attention is a beam of light, like a searchlight, that starts in the middle of you and beams out to whichever part of your body that I mention.

Now bring your attention to the very centre of yourself, the middle of your mind. For each person this is different. For some people it may be in the middle of your head. For some it may be in the middle of your heart, for others it may be another part of your body; there is no right or wrong: wherever this place is for you, take yourself there now. Now bring your beaming light of attention up to the top of your head, to the very tip of your body, the top of your scalp. Focus on the sensations on the top of your scalp, and now sweep your attention down your scalp, slowly and gently. Notice the sensations on your scalp, around the sides, the front of your scalp, the back.

Now notice the skin on your forehead, notice the back of your head at your hairline, the back of your neck, your right ear, your right earlobe, your left earlobe, your forehead, your right eyebrow, your left eyebrow, your eyelashes as they rest on your cheeks, the cheekbones, your nose, the sensation of air around each nostril as you breathe in, and out, the top of your lip, your bottom lip, your jaw line, right and left, and your chin.

Now move that beam of light down as you focus on your throat and the back of the neck. Now your right shoulder, the top of your shoulder from the neck to the tip of your shoulder, your right arm pit, the lower side of your right upper arm, the outer side of your right upper arm, and then the sides of that arm, your elbow, the crease of your elbow. Your right forearm, upper, lower, outer, inner forearm. Your right hand. Notice the palm of your hand, the back of your hand, your thumb, forefinger, middle finger, ring finger, little finger. The whole of your right hand, the whole of your forearm, the whole of your upper arm, your whole right arm and shoulder.

Now move that beam of light down as you focus on your throat and the back of the neck. Now your left shoulder, the top of your shoulder from the neck to the tip of your shoulder, your left arm pit, the lower side of your left upper arm, the outer side of your left upper arm, and then the sides of that arm, your elbow, the crease of your elbow. Your left forearm, upper, lower, outer, inner forearm. Your left hand. Notice the palm of your hand, the back of your hand, your thumb, forefinger, middle finger, ring finger, little finger. The whole of your left hand, the whole of your forearm, the whole of your upper arm, your whole left arm and shoulder.

Now bring your attention to your chest. Notice the sensations in your chest. Move your attention down to your upper belly, your lower belly, the groin area. Now back up to the back side of your body, your neck, your right shoulder blade and upper back, your left shoulder blade and upper back, your middle back, lower back, right buttock, left buttock. Your whole torso.

Notice the sensations of your upper thigh, the top of your right thigh, the bottom of your right thigh, the sides of the thigh. Notice the knee, the back of the knee, your right shin, your right calf muscle, the back of your lower leg, the sides of your lower leg, your ankle, top, sides, back. Your heel, the arch of your foot, the ball of your foot, and now your right toes, big toe, second toe, middle toe, fourth toe, little toe, the whole of your right foot, the whole of your right lower leg, the whole of your right upper leg, the whole of your right leg.

Notice the sensations of your upper thigh, the top of your left thigh, the bottom of your left thigh, the sides of the thigh. Notice the knee, the back of the knee, your left shin, your left calf muscle, the back of your lower leg, the sides of your lower leg, your ankle, top, sides, back. Your heel, the arch of your foot, the ball of your foot, and now your left toes, big toe, second toe, middle toe, fourth toe, little toe, the whole of your left foot, the whole of your left lower leg, the whole of your leg upper leg, the whole of your left leg.

And now bring your attention to the whole of your lower body, the whole of your upper body, including your head and scalp, and now bring the whole of your body into your attention. Notice all of your body at once.

Now gently deepen your breathing. Wiggle your fingers and toes. We are going to end your awareness practice now. Open your eyes, smile to the world and gently thank yourself for giving your brain this wonderful opportunity to grow.

Positive Personality Adjectives

Adventurous	Enthusiastic	Proud
Affectionate	Fair	Quick-witted
Ambitious	Forgiving	Quiet
Articulate	Friendly	Rational
Artistic	Funny	Reliable
Careful	Generous	Reserved
Cheerful	Gentle	Serious
Compassionate	Helpful	Shy
Considerate	Honest	Silly
Courageous	Imaginative	Sincere
Courteous	Inventive	Studious
Creative	Kind	Sympathetic
Curious	Loyal	Thoughtful
Dependable	Mischievous	Tolerant
Determined	Neat	Tidy
Easy-going	Persistent	Trusting
Empathic	Polite	Wise
Energetic	Practical	

APPENDIX III

Bringing the Five Senses into Awareness

Take some time to settle yourself into your chair.

Sit with both feet on the floor, eyes gently closed or looking into the middle distance.

Rest your hands on your lap, or your forearms on the arms of the chair – whichever is more comfortable.

Start to become aware of your breath. Notice the in breath…and the out breath…

Become aware of being in your body.

Notice the feeling of your feet on the floor…the chair under your thighs, supporting you…the clothes on your skin…the light brush of air on your hands and face.

(Pause)

Next, become aware of your sense of taste. Notice the sensation of taste inside your mouth. It is okay just to notice the sensations…no need to label them.

(Pause)

Next, become aware of your sense of smell, what you can smell… Open your awareness to the aromas around you…again, not labelling so much as noticing…

(Pause)

And now become aware of your sense of sight. Whether your eyes are open or closed, take in what you can see…the colour, shapes, light, shade…

(Pause)

And now begin to become aware of what you can hear. First, notice the sounds closest to you, the sounds in the room. Next, open your awareness to the sounds a little way away, in the middle distance…noticing sounds… Next, begin to be aware of the sounds in the distance…the sounds coming from far away…and then become aware of the silence that exists in between the sounds…

Now gently deepen your breathing. Wiggle your fingers and toes. We are going to end your awareness practice now. Open your eyes, smile to the world and gently thank yourself for giving your brain this wonderful opportunity to grow.

Daily Energy Account Form

Date:			
Energy Account			
Withdrawals		**Deposits**	
Activity/Experience	**(0–100)**	**Activity/Experience**	**(0–100)**
Total:		Total:	
Closing Balance (Debit/Credit):			
If necessary, what can I do tomorrow to compensate?			
How can I schedule more energy-infusing activities into my day?			

Progressive Muscle Relaxation

Being able to relax when we need to relax is one of the most liberating skills to learn in life. A calm brain is a smarter brain, so we tend to make better choices when we are relaxed. Life is more enjoyable when we are relaxed. A highly effective way to learn to relax, if the skill proves elusive, is to learn the relaxation method of Progressive Muscle Relaxation (PMR). PMR involves sequentially tensing and relaxing each of the major muscle groups in the body in turn. Like any other skill, it takes some time to learn, so please do not be deceived by the simplicity of the instructions. It looks simple but it can be difficult to stay focussed. We highly recommend staying with the practice even when you do not feel like it, in order to reap the amazing benefits of this skill. By 'staying with the practice' we mean scheduling 15–20 minutes of PMR daily for at least two weeks. Whilst this may seem a long time, we find that many people start to really enjoy the periods of relaxation in their day and start to wonder how they ever coped with life without these periods. If PMR is not for you, you will know after two weeks and you may wish to try a different relaxation method, for example meditation, yoga or yoga nidra, hypnosis for relaxation, Qi Gong or Tai Chi.

If you are not used to tuning in to being in your body you may start to notice sensations that you do not like. If this happens, please try to stay with the practice whilst gently reassuring yourself that you are safe, you are in complete control of your experience. Try to remain an observer to any uncomfortable sensations that may arise. Of course, if the sensation that is bringing discomfort is a result of the position you are in during RPM, find ways to make yourself more physically comfortable for your PMR. For example, lie down, instead of staying seated. If lying down with lower back pain, place a large pillow under your knees or lie with your knees bent and touching, with your feet at hips width.

Take some time now to settle yourself into a comfortable position. You may choose to sit in a comfortable armchair or to lie down on the floor, on a mat, or on your bed. Make sure that you are warm. The body will cool down during this relaxation but it is important that you remain comfortable. If you choose to lie down, please ensure that you place a pillow underneath your head to support your neck and head. Also ensure that your lower back is comfortable. Sometimes people find that it is helpful to place a second pillow under the knees to take the pressure from the lower back.

Take these next few moments to check into your body to see if there are any other minor adjustments that you can make to make your body even 10 per cent more comfortable.

Consciously take in a deep breath through the nose, filling the lungs with oxygen, hold the breath for 3 seconds, and then gently and slowly release the breath through the nose. Take in another deep breath through the nose, hold your breath for 2 seconds, then gently release the breath through the nose.

We are now going to start a wonderful relaxation strategy to bring calm and a sense of ease to the body. Thank yourself for giving yourself this time to practise relaxation, knowing that in the next few minutes there is nothing that you need to do, no one that you need to see or avoid – this is a time just for you, to practice relaxation.

In progressive muscle relaxation, we mindfully bring tension into one part of the body only, and then mindfully release the tension from that part of the body. We do this in timing with our breath. Concentrate on taking a breath in whilst you are bringing tension into the part of the body I have labelled. On the release of tension, concentrate on releasing the breath at the same time. Whilst holding tension in one part of the body as requested, focus on relaxing the other parts of the body at the same time.

Hands

First, bring your attention to your hands. On the in-breath, squeeze your hands into fists. Bring the tension into your body. Now hold the tension in your hands while you hold the breath for 3 more seconds. 1, 2, 3. Now release the breath and the tension at the same time, whilst counting to 3. 1, 2, 3. Feel the tension leave your hands. Feel softness where there was tension. Wonderful, well done.

Arms

I want you now to bring your attention to your arms. Whilst taking in a breath and counting to 3, hold your arms out in front of you, bringing tension into the arms to make both the forearms and upper arms stiff like a board. Hold the tension for a count of 3. 1, hold the tension…2, squeeze…3. Now release the tension from the arms and release the breath at the same time whilst counting to 3. 1, 2, 3. Feel softness in the arms where before they were tense and stiff. Allow softness and stillness to be in the arms now.

Shoulders and neck

Now, whilst relaxing the rest of your body, bring your attention to your shoulders and neck. Whilst taking in a breath and counting to 3, squeeze your shoulders toward your ears, bringing tension into the neck to the level that is comfortable for you. Hold and squeeze for 3. 1, squeeze…2, hold…3. Now release the tension and the breath at the same time whilst counting to 3. 1, 2, 3. Well done. Welcome the ease and softness into your shoulders and neck.

Face

Now, whilst relaxing the rest of your body, bring your attention to your face. Take in a breath, screw up your face into a grimace, bringing tension into all the small muscles of your face, including your tongue and jaw. Hold for 3. 1, squeeze…2, hold…3. Now release the tension and the breath at the same time whilst counting to 3. 1, 2, 3. Feel the jaw and facial muscles soften and relax. Wonderful work.

Stomach

Moving down the body, bring your attention to your stomach. We tend to hold a lot of tension in our stomachs. If you know this is true for you, I recommend that you gently place loving hands on your stomach for this part of the exercise. Placing loving hands on your stomach will allow you to release even more tension. Whilst taking in a breath and counting to 3, contract your stomach muscles together, drawing your energy in as if you were about to lift your legs off the floor using only your stomach muscles. Hold the tension to a level that is comfortable for you. Hold and squeeze for a count of 3. 1, squeeze…2, hold…3. Now gently release the tension in your stomach and release the breath at the same time whilst counting to 3. 1, 2, 3. Well done. If you have your hands on your stomach, you may gently move them to the floor, or the arms of the chair now. Relax the whole of your body, let go of all tension.

Buttocks

Now, bring your attention to your buttocks. Whilst taking in a breath and counting to 3, squeeze the cheeks of your buttocks together, bringing tension to the cheeks of your buttocks. Hold for 3. 1, squeeze your buttocks…2, hold the tension…3. Now release the tension and the breath at the same time whilst counting to 3. 1, 2, 3. Good.

Legs

Now, whilst relaxing the rest of your body, bring your attention to your legs – the whole length of the legs at once. Whilst taking in a breath and counting to 3, bring tension into the whole of your legs. To do so, focus on tensing up the calf and the thigh muscles in both legs at the same time. Hold for a count of 3. 1, squeeze…2, hold the tension…3. Now release the tension and the breath at the same time whilst counting to 3. 1, 2, 3. Good work. Notice the softness in the muscles of your legs as you let go of all the tension.

Feet

Take a moment to relax the whole of your body. Now bring your attention to your feet. Whilst taking in a breath and counting to 3, bring tension into your feet to a level that is comfortable for you. Squeezing the toes downward toward the heels can be one way of bringing tension into the feet. Squeeze and hold for 3 with the breath. 1, squeeze…2, hold…3. Now release the tension and the breath at the same time whilst counting to 3. 1, 2, 3. Relax the feet. Allow them to rest on the floor, or, if you are lying down, to flop to each side.

Whole body

Now, we are going to tense the whole body at once. Draw in the breath and, whilst counting to 3, bring tension into the whole of your body at once. Ball up your fists, straighten your arms and legs, screw up your face into a grimace, ball up your feet, squeeze your shoulders toward your ears, and squeeze your stomach and buttock muscles together. Squeeze and hold the tension for a count of 3. 1, squeeze all parts of your body…2, hold…3. Now release the tension and the breath at the same time whilst counting to 3. 1, 2, 3. Excellent work.

Now it is time to simply relax and let go of all the tension that has been brought into the body. Gently allow your awareness to touch on each part of the body as I name that part. As your awareness gently touches each part of the body, say in your own mind 'Relax, let go.' Hands…arms…shoulders…neck…face…and jaw… stomach…buttocks…legs…feet… The whole of your body, just relaxing. Give yourself permission to stay in this position for a few moments. This is relaxation. It is a different state to muscle tension. Relaxed muscles give a message to our brain to be calm. Remember this feeling of relaxation, it is yours whenever you need it. The more you practice relaxation the more quickly, comfortably and easily you will be able to relax. Learning to relax is a skill that is worth learning. Remember it is a practice, not a performance. The mind may judge what you are doing here. If you notice your mind is judging you or what you are doing, just notice and let that go. Bring your mind back the sensation of rest, softness, relaxation in the muscles. A relaxed body is a relaxed mind.

Now gently, begin to wiggle your fingers and toes. Gently move your head from side to side. Do what you need to do to bring energy back into your body: stretch, sigh, yawn. If you are lying down, roll your body to the side. Allow yourself to rest in a foetal position for a moment before gently sitting up. Gently open your eyes, and thank yourself for giving your mind and body this beautiful practice. Gently now move through the rest of the activities of your day, consciously allowing yourself to relax when tension starts to come back into the body. Have a beautiful, relaxed day.

Relaxation for Self-awareness

Seat yourself comfortably in the chair. If you wish to, close your eyes. Closing your eyes can be helpful to allow the mind to focus on what is being said. Start to become aware of your breath. You may breathe through your nose or your mouth. Notice which, and feel the sensation of the air entering your body, filling your lungs, and then leaving your body. You may wish to control your breathing by increasing the breaths you take into deep ones that fill your lungs, or you may wish to simply observe your breathing. Both are just perfect. As you are focusing on the breath, you are aware of sounds in the room and particularly my voice. As you relax in the chair, I am going to describe a scene that you can go to in your imagination.

I want you to imagine that you are in a time capsule and about to travel back into the past. Enter the time capsule and begin to go back in time to a place where you felt very, very happy about something you did, an achievement, a success. It is good to stop at the first memory you have when there was a success that you achieved, or were a part of, and you felt really good about yourself. There may have been someone else there who was important to you, and that person shared with you how proud they were about your achievement. Take yourself to that time now.

When you have a picture in your mind of a time when you felt happy and successful, stay with that memory for a bit. Imagine that you are that age now, the very age you were when you experienced that delicious experience of success. Begin to feel again the experience. Take your time to expand the memory in your mind, imagine your surrounds, see them vividly in your mind, the colours, the quality of the light, who was there, what they were saying. If someone was there, imagine seeing them now, and imagine them saying something really nice to you about what you have achieved. Feel again the temperature of the scene, experience what you can smell and hear. Now take yourself inside your body and experience how it feels to be so happy, to feel achievement, success, and fulfilment. Experience the sensation in your body, in your legs and arms, your stomach, your heart. Say to yourself, 'Yes, I did it. Well done! I have succeeded at something I know is important. I am happy and proud.' Reflect on your key strengths and say them to yourself. Know that your success is tied to you, to your abilities and qualities. You always have these strengths in you, no one can take them away, they make up a crucial part of you. And whenever you wish to, you can draw on these strengths and experience success, happiness and fulfilment.

Now, slowly begin to experience your body in the room, and as you come back to that awareness, bring the experience of success with you. Wiggle your fingers and toes. Notice your breath. Open your eyes.

Time Machine Activity

Seat yourself comfortably in the chair. If you wish to, close your eyes. Closing your eyes can be helpful to allow the mind to focus on what is being said. Start to become aware of your breath. You may breathe through your nose or your mouth. Notice which, and feel the sensation of the air entering your body, filling your lungs, and then leaving your body. You may wish to control your breathing by increasing the breaths you take into deep ones that fill your lungs, or you may wish to simply observe your breathing. Both are just perfect. As you are focusing on the breath, you are aware of sounds in the room and particularly my voice. As you relax in the chair, I am going to describe a scene that you can go to in your imagination.

I want you to imagine that you are in a time capsule and about to travel ten years into the future. Enter the time capsule and begin to go forward in time to a place where you feel very, very happy about something you have accomplished, an achievement, a success. Bring the success into your mind vividly. There will be people there who are important to you, and new people that you have not yet met who are so happy to celebrate your achievement with you. Take yourself to that time and place now.

When you have a picture in your mind of your future success, stay with that image for a while. Begin to feel the experience. Take your time to expand the image in your mind, imagine your surrounds, see them vividly in your mind, the colours, the quality of the light.

Imagine where you are living at this stage in your life, who you are living with. Imagine the work or study that you are doing. Imagine the people who are in your life; who is important to you.

Bring yourself back to the scene of your celebration. Who is there? What are they saying? See a person who loves and cares about you, and imagine them saying something really nice to you about what you have achieved. Imagine there are new people there, also congratulating you and smiling at you with affection and love and caring. Feel the temperature of the scene, experience what you can smell and hear. Now take yourself inside your body and experience how it feels to be so happy, to feel achievement, success, and fulfilment. Experience the sensation in your body, in your legs and arms, your stomach, your heart. Say to yourself, 'Yes, I did it. Well done! I have succeeded at something I know is important. I am happy and proud.'

Bring to mind your key strengths and say them to yourself. Know that your success is tied to you, to your abilities and qualities. You always have these strengths in you, no one can take them away, they make up a crucial part of you. And whenever you wish to, you can draw on these strengths and experience success, happiness, and fulfilment.

Now, slowly begin to experience your body in the room, and as you come back to that awareness, bring the experience of success with you. Wiggle your fingers and toes. Notice your breath. Open your eyes.

Mood Diary Dimensions

HAPPY	RELAXED	AFFECTION	SMART
HAPPY / HAPPY 20 19 18 17 16 15 14 13 12 11 10 9 8 7 6 5 4 3 2 1 0 SAD / SAD	RELAXED / RELAXED 20 19 18 17 16 15 14 13 12 11 10 9 8 7 6 5 4 3 2 1 0 ANXIOUS / ANXIOUS	AFFECTION / AFFECTION 20 19 18 17 16 15 14 13 12 11 10 9 8 7 6 5 4 3 2 1 0 ANGER / ANGER	SMART / SMART 20 19 18 17 16 15 14 13 12 11 10 9 8 7 6 5 4 3 2 1 0 STUPID / STUPID
SAD	ANXIOUS	ANGER	STUPID

Glossary

Alexipersona A limited vocabulary of words to describe the different types and characteristics of personality, both in oneself and in others.

Alexithymia A diminished vocabulary of words to describe emotions; this includes one's own emotions as well as the emotions of other people.

Cognitive Relating to the mental processes involved in acquiring knowledge and understanding through thought, experience and the senses. These processes encompass attention, memory, judgement and evaluation, comprehension, reasoning and problem solving, and decision making.

Cognitive restructuring The process of learning to identify, challenge and replace irrational or illogical thought or beliefs.

Dyskinesia An abnormality or impairment of voluntary movement.

Dysthymia A mood disorder with similar cognitive, emotional and physical characteristics as depression. However, the symptoms are generally milder, and tend to be longer lasting.

Endocrine system The collection of glands that secrete hormones into the circulatory system.

Executive function A set of cognitive abilities that includes attention, inhibition, memory and flexible thinking, as well as reasoning, problem solving, planning, organizing and time management.

Generalization The ability to transfer knowledge, behaviour and thinking to different situations.

Hypomanic episode A period of hypomania that may be of concern due to the intensity of the mood state.

Learning profile An analysis and description of a person's learning abilities and difficulties.

Negative reinforcement The psychological process whereby the rate of a specific behaviour or thought increases because an unpleasant event or stimulus is removed or prevented from happening; e.g. a girl tidies her room in order to end her mother nagging.

Neuro-transmitter A chemical 'messenger' that enables or inhibits the transmission of signals between neurones (nerve cells) in the brain.

Neurotypical A term originally created by those with autism to describe people who are not on the autism spectrum. It is now used to describe people who have a 'typical' neurology.

Schema A pattern of thought or behaviour that organizes categories of information and the relationships among those categories. People use schemata (plural) to organize their current knowledge, and provide a framework for future understanding.

Acknowledgements

We would like to express our appreciation to those who contributed to the development of this CBT programme and self-help book:

The original group participants, for their invaluable advice on aspects of the programme that needed further explanation and those aspects that could be edited.

Dawn Sheahan, Tony's personal assistant, for the considerable amount of time and energy spent on the design and production of the original CBT programme, and on the typing of numerous drafts of the book.

William Attwood, Maja Toudal, Rachael Harris and Damian Santomauro, for their thoughtful insights and commentary on the original manuscript.

Sarah Attwood, for correcting and improving several versions of the text, and copyediting the final manuscript.

Adrian Kelly and Robert and Beverlee Garnett, for their unending inspiration, belief and support.

Index